Digital Forensics

Digital Forensics

Digital Evidence in Criminal Investigation

Angus M. Marshall
University of Teesside, UK

WILEY-BLACKWELL

A John Wiley & Sons, Ltd., Publication

This edition first published 2008
© 2008 John Wiley & Sons, Ltd

Wiley-Blackwell is an imprint of John Wiley & Sons, formed by the merger of Wiley's global
Scientific, Technical and Medical business with Blackwell Publishing.

Registered office.
John Wiley & Sons Ltd, The Atrium, Southern Gate, Chichester, West Sussex, PO19 8SQ, UK

Other Editorial Offices:
9600 Garsington Road, Oxford, OX4 2DQ, UK
111 River Street, Hoboken, NJ 07030-5774, USA

For details of our global editorial offices, for customer services and for information about how to
apply for permission to reuse the copyright material in this book please see our website at
www.wiley.com/wiley-blackwell

Library of Congress Cataloging-in-Publication Data

Marshall, Angus M.
    Digital forensics : digital evidence in criminal investigation / Angus M. Marshall.
        p. ; cm.
    Includes bibliographical references and index.
    ISBN 978-0-470-51774-1 (cloth)
    1. Digital electronics.   2. Forensic engineering.   I. Title.
    [DNLM: 1. Forensic Medicine–methods.   2. Computers.   3. Forensic
Medicine–instrumentation.   4. Internet.   W 626.5 M367d 2008]
    TK7868.D5M3215 2008
    363.25–dc22

                                                                        2008033258

ISBN: 9780470517741 (HB)
ISBN: 9780470517758 (PB)

A catalogue record for this book is available from the British Library.

Typeset in 11/15pt Minion by Aptara Inc., New Delhi, India.
Printed in Singapore by Markono Print Media Pte Ltd
First impression – 2008

Contents

Preface

A small auto-biography

For most of my life, I've been fascinated by computers. At school, one of my maths teachers, Mr. Brindle, had a Commodore PET (Personal Electronic Translator) which formed the nucleus of a computer club.

A gang of us would gather at lunchtimes and after school, trying to devise new games and solve interesting problems. Soon, an Apple][was acquired and the club members had to relearn programming for this strange new creature. We even managed to get access to the holy mainframe (a DEC-20) at our local college and many evenings were spent exploring the capabilities of this magnificent beast.

Around this time, the Computer Misuse Act and the first Data Protection Act were being drafted and brought into legislation, defining specific offences relating to inappropriate and unauthorised use of computer systems. The first mobile phones started to appear and CD-players were a "must-have" gadget. Companies such as Commodore, Sinclair and Acorn enjoyed huge success with their home computers and Apple and IBM started production of personal computers aimed at businesses.

I was supposed to be a physicist, but an early introduction to the possibilities of computer networks led me into some experimentation with primitive "hacking" – nearly ruining my attempts to gain a BSc. Eventually, I did graduate with a degree in Computer Studies and Microsystems by forcing myself to concentrate on the challenge of getting hardware and software to work in harmony. My first real academic research dealt with the creation of neural networks on parallel processing systems, but I was developing more of an interest in a thing called the "Internet", which seemed, to me, to have great potential for information sharing and creating online communities. An emerging Internet service called the "World Wide Web" seemed to be a very accessible way of using the Internet, and combining it with my other passion (proper sports cars) led to a few years of collaboration with the Morgan Motor Company, where they gained a WWW presence, and my team gained a better understanding of how people navigate web sites.

Around 1992, I first became aware of the existence of "Forensic Computing" as an emerging discipline, concentrating on how data could be recovered from computers for use in criminal investigations.

For the following 10 years, or so, I continued as computer science lecturer in a number of British universities, finally landing at the Centre for Internet Computing in Scarborough where I was able to introduce some aspects of forensic computing into the curriculum, in the guise of modules dealing with computer security. I was also fortunate enough to have a colleague who shared some of my interests, and discovered that we made a good research team. So, we began writing and publishing papers, which were accepted by the general forensic science community to such an extent that it was suggested that I should register with the National Crime Faculty as an expert adviser on Internet activities.

Then, in 2003, I received a call from a police force asking if I could help them with a missing person enquiry. Soon, it transpired that we were dealing with a murder enquiry, and computer-originated evidence turned out to be almost essential in establishing patterns of behaviour and interests for the victim and more than one suspect.

Since then, I have acted as an expert witness for prosecution and defence in all manner of cases from fraud, through copyright violation to distribution of illegal images of children. The cases are always serious, but the work is never boring – with new challenges presented every time.

Now, I am a member of the Forensic and Crime Scene Sciences team at the University of Teesside where I am lucky enough to work with experts from a huge range of other disciplines.[1] My own group (Digital Evidence) is expanding steadily and we provide material for all of the forensic and crime scene science courses in our school. I also act as an external examiner and

---

[1] Some of whom do their experiments in buckets.

adviser/consultant for other universities, and maintain links with business and industry wherever possible.

About this book

The world is full of digital devices. Without them, society as we know it would probably collapse. As a result, even the most innocuous device may contain information which is relevant in a criminal investigation. This book is intended to help investigators assess the potential of digital evidence sources, evaluate the huge and ever-changing range of technologies available, and introduce some of the main principles of digital evidence examination.

It does not go into excessive low-level detail of how files are deleted in the NTFS MFT, for example, but concentrates more on how those involved in criminal investigations can consider the potential of digital devices as sources of evidence; suggest possible lines of enquiry which can assist the investigator and, I hope, help them to understand the principles behind some of the more technical aspects of digital evidence examination.

Finally, an apology. To all my colleagues in the forensic science world: I know that "forensic" is an adjective relating to debating or courts and should never be used as a noun or, worse yet, a verb... but sometimes editors win arguments.

Angus Marshall

Acknowledgments

The list of people who need to be thanked for their support in the production of this book is immense, but a few in particular deserve special thanks:

- Fiona and the team at Wiley: for tolerating my Adams-like attitude to deadlines.

- Allen Clarkson: for reading drafts and passing comments – always helpfully.

- Brian Tompsett and Natasha Semmens: my regular research partners and co-investigators in the Cyberprofiling project. Without their support, some of the ideas in this book could never have existed.

- Colleagues at the University of Teesside: who have taught me far too much about forensic and crime scene sciences and influenced my approach to casework.

- My students: for making me think much harder than I wanted to, sometimes. I hope I've done the same to you.

- My parents: for giving me a second chance all those years ago.

And, most importantly, my wife Shirley, who supported and encouraged me throughout this whole process.

List of Tables

List of Figures

1

Introduction

The field of digital evidence, aka Forensic Computing, is unlike most other forensic sciences because the nature of the material under examination is determined, largely, by human ingenuity. Rather than looking for traces of material deposited by physical or biological entities, which tend to develop and evolve slowly, we deal with technology which is updated, enhanced and even created at an alarming rate.

Since the 1960s, the rate of development of digital technology has held true to Moore's law [32], which originally proposed that the density of transistors on a given area of silicon would double approximately every 18 months. Since the start of the 21st century, the rate has slowed slightly, but we still see a doubling in density every two years.

This means that a modern mobile phone can contain more processing power and storage capacity than the computers which NASA used to send man to the moon. In a device a fraction of the size. At a much lower price. And easier to use. With greater reliability. And a smaller power supply.

1.1 Key developments

The time when only nerds or geeks[1] were interested in computers is long gone. Advances in computer usability have led to the development of digital

---

[1] A geek is a nerd with social skills, and an extrovert geek looks at *your* shoes when he/she is talking to you.

Digital Forensics: Digital Evidence in Criminal Investigation Angus M. Marshall
© 2008 John Wiley & Sons, Ltd

devices which are no longer the sole preserve of the white-coated "high priests" of computing (once known as the programmers and operators), but have become accessible to everyone capable of holding a mouse or using a keyboard.

Increasing dependence on computers can, arguably, be traced back to the late 1970s and early 1980s with the development of machines such as the Apple][, Lisa and Macintosh; Sinclair ZX81 and Spectrum; Commodore Vic20, 64 and Amiga and, finally, the IBM Personal Computer [8].

The IBM PC, with its standardised low-cost hardware, simple Microsoft Disc Operating System (PC-DOS or MS-DOS) and the backing of the world's largest computer manufacturer, resulted in a host of imitators and compatible machines targeted mainly at business.

It seems that Pournelle's law[2] was perceived to be true in business. The creation of low-cost machines that allowed users to perform common computing tasks on their desktops, without having to wait for time on the company mainframe or mini-computer, led to the first steps towards pervasive computing: "computing anywhere and everywhere".

The success of these IBM-compatible PCs with Microsoft operating systems and applications created a de-facto standard, never before seen, which allowed free exchange of data and information between systems, people and organisations, thus eliminating one of the biggest barriers to information exchange.

Standardisation of software and data created opportunities for "paper-less offices", where every member of staff had access to computing resources on the desktop – often linked to a local area network – connecting machines within an office or building for even greater resource sharing and efficiency.

Meanwhile, since the 1960s, work had been progressing on what we know today as the Internet [43]. This wide area network began life as an academic project designed to allow data sharing between distant sites, but in a way which allowed the network to be scaled up to include millions of machines. Again, this created a de-facto international standard for networking through the creation of an easy to use system which allowed developers to

---

[2]"At least one CPU per user" – Jerry Pournelle, science fiction author and BYTE columnist, 1978.

add new features without compromising the existing network. In effect, the Internet provides a global "road network" which is capable of carrying any type of traffic which can be devised.

Prior to 1989, however, the Internet was largely the preserve of the technically minded, mostly because of the huge number of incompatible applications which existed on it. Tim Berners-Lee, a British physicist working at CERN, proposed a new information management system [5] for CERN to counter the problems of information loss, damage and confusion which the organisation was suffering at the time.

The proposal defined an information sharing system which allowed disparate information systems to be linked together via a common interface based around the concept of HyperText [4].[3] In a HyperText system, the user can navigate around the text by activsting links, which jump to other pieces of text. Berners-Lee's innovation was to allow these links to reference documents and even applications external to the current document. In this way, the World Wide Web as we know it was born, with a single consistent interface to a range of different applications. Arguably, this is the single most important innovation in information systems in the 20th century. It has certainly led to the widespread adoption of Internet services as a part of everyday life.

Alongside, and slightly behind, the developments in desktop computing and internetworking, the continual shrinking of components created opportunities for smaller devices to be created. In the 1980s we saw the creation of the first analogue mobile telephony networks, with a proper launch in the UK in 1982. Although the devices in use were bulky with very limited battery life (typically a few hours), poor network coverage and susceptible to interference and eavesdropping, they were well-received and became essential tools for modern business. 1982[4] also saw the launch of the compact disc (CD) by Philips, setting a new standard for audio and data storage. The thirst for increased capacity in this convenient disc format led to the later creation of the Digital Versatile Disc (DVD) and the current battles over High-Definition disc standards.

---

[3]The term HyperText was coined around 1965 by Ted Nelson, but the concept is older.
[4]A very good year – it also saw the launch of the author's favourite car: the Lotus Excel.

By the 1990s, the GSM[5] [18] standard had been developed for digital mobile telephone networks, providing better quality and better use of the available networks where it was implemented. Continued improvements in technology meant that digital handsets had shrunk in size to become devices which could fit into a briefcase or pocket, with longer battery life and lower cost.

The Internet and the existence of a workable digital telecommunications network, combined with increasingly powerful low-cost devices, also created a desire to distribute more complex data in the form of music, photographs and video. Unfortunately, although the communications technologies were effective, they had not been designed with real-time high-quality audio and video in mind. As a result, it became necessary to develop compression methods such as MPEG [33] which would allow acceptable quality content to be delivered over low-bandwidth connections. The same technology is currently being used for broadcast digital television and is used to allow multiple digital channels to occupy the same bandwidth as a single analogue channel (although the analogue and digital signals cannot be present at the same time). Inadvertently, the MPEG2 standard for digital video had a major impact on the music industry through the creation of a new standard for digital audio – MP3 (MPEG2 layer 3).

The 1990s also saw some major changes in operating systems. Microsoft finally released its "Chicago" software, better known as Windows 95, setting a new baseline for the IBM-compatible world. This included networking in a format which was relatively easy to set up, and considerably easier than the previous Windows 3.11 and Windows for Workgroups systems, which had relied on support being provided by their underlying DOS. Developments of Windows 95 strengthened network and hardware support through Windows 98 and ME until the "home" platform converged with Microsoft's professional operating system (Windows NT) to create Windows XP and, at the start of the 21st century, Windows Vista.

Most recently, a new development in wired telecommunications has driven down the cost of high-performance internetworking to the point where it has become affordable for domestic users. Broadband xDSL

---

[5]Global System for Mobile Communications.

technology, in the form, mainly, of ADSL (Asymmetric Digital Subscriber Line), offers a high-speed digital connection using existing telephone wiring. It offers an always-on connection, for those who want it, and allows consumers to receive more complex, "richer" content, in the form of video and other media, than was previously possible using slow dial-up connections. The increased speed also means that it has become properly possible for someone to work at home as efficiently as they could in an office. The network connection to their home computer is not as fast as the one they would have in the corporate network, but the speed is sufficient for them to access core corporate services such as e-mail.

1.2 Digital devices in society

The result of 40 years of innovation, as outlined above, has been a move towards an increasingly technology-dependent society. It is rare to find anyone who does not have access to some form of computing device, be it in a vehicle (engine management in a modern car), for personal entertainment (MP3 music player, CD player, DVD player etc.), personal communications (mobile telephone), personal computing or lifestyle management (Personal Digital Assitants and smartphones).

Individuals depend on digital technology to manage their personal financial affairs, ensure that goods are in shops for them to purchase and to schedule transport and other activities efficiently. We use mobile phones to communicate, wherever we happen to be, laptop/notebook computers and PDAs to work in any location and the Internet for communications, entertainment and business 24 hours a day, 7 days a week.

From a situation where activities were generally constrained to the immediate local geographic area, we have evolved into a society which operates globally but carries out activities locally. People never actually have to meet or even speak directly to each other, but can interact via e-mail, chatrooms and online ecommerce systems. Even in the preparation of this book, there has been only one face-to-face meeting. All other discussion, negotiation etc. has been carried out using online systems.

Business, industry and commerce are now almost completely dependent on digital technology as a core part of their activities. Without the systems responsible for accepting and processing orders, controlling stock, issuing invoices and managing financial transactions, most businesses would start to suffer a cash-flow crisis within a matter of days.

Honest citizens and criminals alike have equal access to the technology, constrained only by cost and availability. Fortunately, most criminals make use of the technology for mainly legal purposes, but a few choose to use it to support their criminal activities. We shall explore some of the opportunities this creates in later chapters.

No matter how the technology is used, however, it always records some detail of what it is doing and when it is done.

1.3 Technology and culture

Although much technology evolution has been driven by the desire for lower power, higher capacity or greater efficiency, the emergence of consumer-oriented technologies such as Apple's iPod, mobile phones and similar personal devices has resulted in a merging between technology and fashion. In many cases, particularly among the younger members of society, it is no longer enough to have a device, but it is now necessary to have the "right" device. In the same way that people express their common interests and membership of a particular cultural group through clothing and make-up, design features of personal technology can be viewed as an expression of membership of such a group.

Indeed, since the technology has become so personal, possession of the correct device is perceived by some as an essential adjunct to participation in their chosen peer group. Teenagers, especially, seem to view their personal mobile phone as exactly that – a *personal* device which is guarded jealously, perhaps because it gives them a private communications channel to their peers – but only if it is the *right* make and model.

These personal technologies have also changed the way we communicate. There can be few people who have not witnessed the sight of a gang of teenagers walking down the street, heads down, silent apart from the hushed clicking as their thumbs fly across their mobile phone keypads sending and receiving SMS[6] messages.

---

[6]Short Message Service, aka text, aka txt.

1.4 Comment

We seem to have arrived at a time when society is dependent on technology, not so much through need as through choice. We have driven the development of more efficient, cheaper and smaller devices because they seem to make our lives easier. The cost, however, is that we have changed the way we live to such an extent that we must have such devices in order to continue living the way we want to. Those devices, like it or not, monitor almost everything we do and can store pretty accurate records about our movements and interactions. Our technological assistants, therefore, might be viewed as unsleeping witnesses.

2
Evidential Potential of Digital Devices

Because society has embraced technology to such an extent, it is now commonplace to be asked to consider whether or not digital devices may contain some information about any crime which has been committed. Even though the device itself may not have played any part in the activity, its very presence at the scene, or use by one of those involved, often leads to it being a potential source of valuable evidence.

For example, if a child has gone missing we would typically now ask where that child's mobile phone is. A mobile phone, particularly to a younger person, is an essential personal communication tool. They very rarely, if ever, let them out of their sight. If we can find the phone we have either found the person, or found a location where something significant happened to them: i.e. a crime scene.

The next typical question would be about any computers that the child had access to and whether they had personal e-mail accounts. In this case, we are considering who they have been in contact with, and trying to find out if they have arranged a meeting that their parents or guardians are unaware of.

However, before we can ask these questions, we need to think about the general nature of digital devices and the various roles they can perform in human activity and crime in particular.

Digital Forensics: Digital Evidence in Criminal Investigation   Angus M. Marshall
© 2008 John Wiley & Sons, Ltd

2.1 Closed vs. open systems

To start with, we can consider all digital devices to fall into one of two main categories: *closed* or *open*, depending on how they have been used in the past.

2.1.1 Closed systems

From the point of view of a forensic examiner, a *closed* system is any system which has never been connected to the Internet. This means that it has only ever existed as an isolated entity within a controlled and known environment. Any machines to which it has been connected have been closed systems themselves, thus creating a closed network; another form of closed system.

In effect, then, a closed system may consist of multiple smaller systems all of which satisfy the definition of a closed system.

2.1.2 Open systems

An *open* system, by contrast, is any system, no matter how large or small, which has, at some time, had some sort of connection to the Internet. This connection may have been direct (e.g. through connection to a public wireless network at a coffee shop) or indirect (e.g. through the use of a USB memory device which had previously been used in an Internet-connected system). No matter what the form of the connection and how many steps removed, any association with the Internet converts a closed system into an open system.

2.1.3 Why does this matter?

Consider a conventional crime scene. Let's say there's been a suspicious death and a body has been discovered.

If the body is found in a room where all the doors and windows are locked from the inside, we can assume with a fair degree of confidence that anything that happened to the victim must have happened inside that room and that the cause of death may still be present. We can also be fairly sure that any evidence relating to the events in that room will still be there. Because nothing has been allowed to enter or leave the room, we are pretty sure that nothing in there has changed (apart from the condition of the victim) since the room was locked.

If the body is found on a busy high street, however, we know that the evidence is contaminated by the changing environment around it. Fibres, debris, biological material are all being blown around by the wind, shaken off clothing etc.

In effect, a closed digital system is akin to the sealed room. No matter how large the network is, we can always determine its perimeter and identify each and every item in it.

With an open system, though, we have the busy high street scenario. Systems are joining and leaving the Internet every second of every day. New programs are being created, systems are changing state, users are creating different types of traffic and transferring data. The involvement of the Internet, and the fact that it is impossible to accurately record the complete state of the Internet at any time, introduces new opportunities for contamination of our *virtual* crime scene. So, with open systems, we may have a degree of uncertainty in our understanding of the crime scene that we are dealing with.

Open systems, as a general rule, are much richer sources of information about people and their activities, habits and interests. This is because they offer access to the rich world of the Internet, where communication is the main purpose. As a result, any Internet-connected system will typically contain masses of data representing interactions with others on the network.

Closed systems, on the other hand, may have little value as evidence sources in non-computer crime because they tend to be used for just a few tasks and offer no opportunity for outside contact.

2.1.4 Changes in complexity

The change in complexity caused by the involvement of an Internet connection creates added complexity in the investigative process. The examiner may need to look beyond the evidence present in the virtual crime scene and start to consider which external influences may have been involved in depositing material on the device under examination. This goes beyond consideration of the common malware threats such as viruses, Trojan Horses and backdoors to encompass hackers, deliberate attacks and accidental damage too.

2.1.5 Locality of offence

When considering open systems, as defined above, we may need to consider an additional problem for investigators. Where did the activity take place?

Consider the situation where an Eastern-European hacker has decided to attack a British company, but has relayed their network activity through systems in Korea, Japan and America. (Something which is well within the capabilities of any hacker worth the name.)

Where does the attack take place? Is it purely within the UK, where the attacked system is, or is it in Eastern Europe, where the attacker is physically located? Could it, somehow, be taking place in Korea, Japan or America?

This issue, of *locality of offence* [27] is one that can be troublesome for any investigation which involves the Internet. It may not be possible for us to accurately determine which countries are involved in the activity, and if we cannot determine the countries, we cannot determine the applicable legal systems. Without knowing the laws which apply, we cannot clearly identify any offences which may have occurred.

Even where we can identify the countries involved, it may be that local laws do not define the activity under investigation to be illegal. In fact, this is exactly the problem which happened with the "Lovebug" or "I love you" [20] virus which struck in 2000. Eventually, the originator of the virus was traced to the Phillipines, where it transpired that there was no law which dealt with computer misuse of this type.

Without alignment between the legislation in different countries, it can be difficult to reach agreements about investigations which need to cross national boundaries. This can hold true, even if the legislation in the

Table 2.1 Roles played by digital devices

	Witness	Tool	Accomplice	Guardian	Victim
Closed	CW	CT	CA	CG	CV
Open	OW	OT	OA	OG	OV

victim's country allows for someone to be prosecuted for activity outside that country.

2.1.6 Roles played by digital devices

Although digital devices are fairly passive in nature (i.e. they only perform actions in response to instructions received), they exist only to participate in human activities. Thus they can fulfil several of the roles typically found in crime (Table 2.1) no matter whether they are open or closed systems.

Witness

Commonly, a witness is a passive observer of the activity. It has no direct contact with the participants, but may be able to describe the activity, the environmental conditions and the participants with varying levels of detail.

For our purposes, a digital witness is any system which has had the opportunity to observe something related to the incident we are investigating. Examples range from current Closed Circuit Television (CCTV), which records to hard disc, to network management devices which may have records of traffic passing through them.

Of course, not all witnesses are purely witnesses. Some may have had some involvement in the activity as well.

Tool

A tool, in this context, is defined as something which makes the activity easier, but is not essential. It may be a single piece of software, an individual device or a complete network of machines.

Accomplice

Accomplices are those participants who are essential to the success of the activity. Without them, it is virtually impossible to carry out the act. In the human world, accomplices are usually considered to be active participants in the crime, but may be coerced in some way throught threats, bribes etc.

Digital systems, however, have no inherent conception of right and wrong, or understanding of the law. Their participation as accomplices may be the result of direct contact with the criminal, effectively making them a willing participant through behaviour "learned" from regular association with the miscreant. Alternatively, it may occur as a result of some inherent flaw or weakness in their design or configuration. The criminal may exploit this vulnerability directly or by implanting malware (viruses, Trojan Horses etc.), giving the effect of coercion.

Victim

Victim has its usual meaning here. The victim is the target of the attack.

In the context of digital systems, however, it is rare to find a situation where the system itself is the true target. More commonly, an attack on the system is used as a means to attack the corporation and/or human beings associated with it. Thus any evaluation which proposes that a device sits only in the *CV* or *OV* categories should be treated with suspicion. In practice, anything which does sit in either of the *victim* categories should be examined closely to see if it should also be considered to lie within the *accomplice* categories as well.

Guardian

Guardianship is a concept which did not exist in early versions of this model [27, 25].

From work on cyberprofiling [48, 30], however, it is apparent that criminological Routine Activity Theory [10, 9] (which tells us that a crime can only happen when a motivated attacker and a suitable victim are brought together in the absence of an appropriate guardian) has some parallels in the digital world. Further consideration of digital devices reveals that they can perform some of the functions of a guardian and it is appropriate to include that role in the model. The use of this criminological model is examined in more detail in Chapter 9.

2.1.7 Determining roles

Any device may have several of the roles within the activity under investigation, and it has proved useful in the past to draw up a grid, such as the one shown in Table 2.1, to help evaluate the evidential potential of any devices. The higher the involvement in the activity, the greater the value any evidence recovered from a device is likely to have.

In order to carry out an assessment, it is essential to be able to break the incident down into its component parts and then consider which, if any, devices might have been involved in each stage/phase. Once the devices are identified, their roles can be plotted in the grid.

Examples of role determination

Illegal DVD copying There are really only two ways to produce copies of DVDs. The first involves purchasing the necessary equipment and setting up a factory; clearly this is impractical for the type of criminal who intends to produce a small number of DVDs and sell them through car-boot sales or trading on the streets and in pubs.

The second method is far more accessible. For a few hundred pounds, anyone can buy a standard desktop PC from a high street retailer and equip it with additional DVD-writers and software. Using this far cheaper technology, a "low-level" criminal can start production within a few hours.

Clearly, there is one major device in this activity: the PC itself.

Since we have no suggestion that the PC in question has been connected to the Internet at any point, we may start by considering it a closed system.

Table 2.2   Roles a PC plays in DVD copying

	Witness	Tool	Accomplice	Guardian	Victim
Closed	×		×	×	
Open					

Since it is almost impossible to produce the discs without the PC, it must fulfil an accomplice role. Accomplices, however, are also witnesses, and they occupy a prime location close to the incident. Furthermore, DVD technology incorporates a form of copyright protection designed to prevent casual copying, so the PC should also have a role as guardian, although this has been subverted to turn it into a coerced accomplice. This evaluation leads us to the grid in Table 2.2.

The three categories identified (*CW, CA, CG*) give a strong indication that the PC itself is likely to be a rich source of evidence, and that the criminal must have taken some action to break the guardianship in order to turn it into an accomplice.

Of course, if we have an indication that the PC may have been connected to the Internet at some point (e.g. because the criminal has been selling discs online or has been downloading cover artwork to make the copies seem more legitimate), we should promote it from a closed system to an open system and consider the nature of the other activities.

For example, setting up online auctions would add the *OT: Open system Tool* category. In this case it is appropriate to consider the PC as a tool because the Internet activity could have been conducted on any appropriate system.

Murder   It may seem strange to consider the roles of digital devices in an instance of murder but, as has been previously discussed, although they may not be able to conclusively identify the murderer they can contain significant information which has value as forensic intelligence.

Experience tells us that it is less likely that someone is killed by a complete stranger than a family member, friend or other known contact. Therefore, we start with the assumption that the killer and the victim are likely to be known to each other and to have communicated in some way.

In the modern world, it would be common for them to communicate using mobile phones or e-mail, so we need to consider these devices. Immediately, we can start to look for six devices: the victim's mobile phone, the victim's home computer, the victim's work computer, the killer's mobile phone, the killer's work computer and the killer's home computer.

Since we start with little or no clue to the identity of the killer, we will concentrate on the victim's devices.

The mobile phone will have acted as a tool and witness at least, but since it has the potential to connect to the Internet (a common feature of modern mobile phones) we must consider it to be an open system. Thus it lies in the *OT* and *OW* categories.

Similarly, the two computers may have been used for communication between victim and killer so they also fall into the *OT* and *OW* categories.

When/if we determine who the suspect(s) are, their mobile phone(s) and computer(s) will also fall into the *OT* and *OW* categories.

2.2 Evaluating digital evidence potential

The method described above allows us to evaluate the activities in which devices have participated, but it does not yet allow us to identify which devices have greatest evidential potential.

As a rule of thumb, the more categories the device falls into, the greater significance it is likely to have, particularly when those categories lie to the right hand side (*Accomplice, Victim, Guardian*) of the table. This is because these categories tend to represent active participants in the activity, rather than passive components.

Given the murder situation, described above, however – how would we choose which of the devices should be examined first?

Obviously we would like to concentrate on the devices which contain most data of relevance, but this cannot be determined until the devices have been examined.

In this situation, we must think about the nature of the device itself, and how long data are likely to be preserved within it. A general rule, though, is that if the device is battery powered, it is probably going to lose data when the battery goes flat, so it needs to be dealt with *quickly*. At the very least, we need to create an *image* of the device so that its contents can be examined properly at some later time. This process will be discussed in Chapter 4.

No matter which devices we identify, though, it is crucial that they are correctly handled. By far the most common source of problems in digital evidence handling is the establishment and maintenance of the *chain of custody*.

3

Device Handling

Any Crime Scene Investigator, Scenes of Crime Officer, solicitor, barrister or judge will confirm that the establishment of continuity of evidence can be a crucial issue in a criminal trial. If doubt can be cast over the history of any item of evidence, allowing the suggestion that it has been tampered with during an undocumented period in its life, then the value of that item as reliable evidence is diminished. In extreme cases, it can be so compromised as to be ruled inadmissible – causing a case to collapse.

This is particularly true of digital devices as, unlike some other forensic sciences, we cannot "split" them into separate samples for testing using different processes by independent parties. The act of cutting a digital device into pieces tends to stop it working at all.

The Association of Chief Police Officers for England and Wales produces the "Good Practice Guide for Computer Based Electronic Evidence" [2],[1] which lays down four key principles applicable to the handling and processing of digital devices.

These principles are:

Principle 1:
  No action taken by law enforcement agencies or their agents should change data held on a computer or storage media which may subsequently be relied upon in court.

---

[1] The same document includes issues specific to working within Scots law too.

Digital Forensics: Digital Evidence in Criminal Investigation   Angus M. Marshall
© 2008 John Wiley & Sons, Ltd

Principle 2:

In circumstances where a person finds it necessary to access original data held on a computer or on storage media, that person must be competent to do so and be able to give evidence explaining the relevance and the implications of their actions.

Principle 3:

An audit trail or other record of all processes applied to computer-based electronic evidence should be created and preserved. An independent third party should be able to examine those processes and achieve the same result.

Principle 4:

The person in charge of the investigation (the case officer) has overall responsibility for ensuring that the law and these principles are adhered to.

Application of these principles is not restricted to laboratory-based examination, but needs to start as soon as any investigator encounters a digital device. Equally, although the principles make reference to "law enforcement" and "case officer", they should be applied in any type of digital forensics work, substituting "investigative" and "manager" respectively, to give:

Principle 1:

No action taken by *investigative* agencies or their agents should change data held on a computer or storage media which may subsequently be relied upon in court.

Principle 4:

The person in charge of the investigation (the *manager*) has overall responsibility for ensuring that the law and these principles are adhered to.

In essence, all these principles can be summarised in four sentences as:

1. Don't modify anything.

2. If you have to risk modifying something, make sure you know what you are doing.

3. *Record everything you do, in the right order.*

4. Someone must take responsibility for making sure everything that is done is both legal and in accordance with these principles.

Principle 3 is particularly important in combination with Principle 2. If anything is mishandled, only accurate recording of what happened to it can allow the examiner to make allowances for incorrect handling, and perform a proper evaluation of the quality and significance of evidence recovered.

3.1 Seizure issues

It is tempting to assume that all digital devices can be seized as soon as they are identified, but this is not always the case. It would be grossly unfair, and possibly even illegal, for an investigator to seize equipment which is vital to a business as a result of suspicions of the activity of a few employees. Care must be taken to ensure that any seizure is *justified*, *appropriate* and *proportionate*.

Anything to be seized must, demonstrably, have the potential to contain evidence relating to the activity. It must be a major source of material and any problems presented by its seizure must be outweighed by its value in the investigation. Classifying devices using the roles grid (Table 2.1) method described in Chapter 2 is one way of demonstrating that these requirements are satisfied.

3.1.1 Crime scenes

At the time of seizure, it is best to consider the environment to be a crime scene and approach it using conventional crime scene procedures. Care should be taken to minimise disturbance of any items in the vicinity.

In the film versions of Richard Gordon's "Doctor" books [17], the surgeon Sir Lancelot Spratt was wont to say "Eyes first and most, hands next and least, and tongue not at all" about the examination of a patient. This is true of crime scenes too.

Before starting any work, it is vital that a thorough visual inspection is carried out with appropriate use of photographs and note-taking to ensure that nothing has been missed and that all risks have been fully considered.

Quarantine

The first step, however, has to be to establish a quarantine around the suspect equipment, moving everyone away from it to ensure that no-one has the opportunity to tamper with it. This removes the potential for any accusations of evidence being "planted" or for the user/owner to attempt to damage any evidence of which they are aware.

Recording status

Once the equipment has been quarantined, it should be checked to see if it is "live", i.e. showing any signs of having power applied and of software running. Its status should be recorded as completely as possible using sketches, photographs and comprehensive notes which describe exactly what can be seen. The temptation to use one's own knowledge of digital devices should be resisted. For example the phrase "A window in the centre of the screen was headed 'Microsoft Word' and contained the text 'Leave the money under the third oak tree'" may be more useful than "A word processor was running". Not every program tells the truth when it is running.

Screensavers have caused some debate amongst digital evidence practitioners in the past. Should a screensaver be stopped or simply recorded and allowed to run? Current thinking is that, since we cannot know what the "safe" way of stopping the screensaver is, it should be allowed to continue running, even if it starts during the seizure process. It is important to remember that a screensaver is just another program in the device, triggered by a lack of user activity, and that it is capable of running other programs designed to cause damage.

Screensavers can be protected by passwords and other mechanisms. If we do not not know exactly how to stop a screensaver running safely, we should treat it with suspicion and avoid doing anything to change its behaviour.

Networks and communications

It may be obvious that the machine is connected to a communications device such as a network port or modem. In this case, opinion is divided about the best action to take. General advice, though, is that in the absence of specialist assistance, the safest option is usually to disconnect the system from communications devices as quickly as possible, often before the status recording is complete.

However, disconnecting a system from a live network/communications sessions presents some risks.

Firstly, if the system is connected to a co-conspirator in some way, the disconnection of the communications without warning may alert members of the gang to the fact that something untoward has happened. This may give them time to destroy evidence of their own involvement before they have been identified.

Secondly, it is possible for any system to detect loss of communications and commence action ranging from deletion of data to, in theory, triggering an explosive device.

Finally, in the case of mobile phones, switching the phone off to remove it from the network causes the phone to change internal data which might have been useful to the investigation. Mobile phones are a special case and are dealt with in more detail in Chapter 8.

It is better, when at all possible, to seek advice from a specialist about how to deal with live communications, but if this is not possible, accurate recording of the actions taken should allow the laboratory-based digital evidence examiner to account for any anomalies caused by actions taken in the field.

Power

Having conducted and recorded a thorough visual inspection, and dealt with the issue of communications, we can turn to the issue of shutting equipment down. With the exception of portable devices (see Chapter 8), it is recommended that all systems to be seized should be shut down as soon as possible after their discovery.

Using the operating system's (O/S) "shut down" or "halt" command is not a good idea, nor is simply pressing the power button.

We are all taught, almost as soon as we start to use computers, that it is vital to shut them down correctly. In most cases, this means using special commands to ensure that all data have been written to storage devices correctly. Anyone who has ever removed a floppy disc from a drive before the light has gone out, or taken a USB memory device out of a Windows PC without using the "safe remove" option will be aware of just how bad the damage can be. Notwithstanding the potential for damaging storage devices, it is still far more dangerous to shut systems down "cleanly" during seizure for two principle reasons.

Firstly, and perhaps most importantly, the O/S shut down is a software process, potentially made up of several programs. Each one of these may cause data to be written to the storage devices. As soon as this happens, ACPO's first principle has been violated and we have created a problem with the integrity of the devices.

Secondly, the shut-down process may not be the same on all machines. Because shut down is a software process, it can be modified at will by knowledgeable users. They may, if they choose to, plant programs in the process in order to damage evidence – or worse.

So, why not press the power-off button?   In modern systems the power button is actually used as a trigger for the O/S shut-down process. Even though pressing it for 10 seconds (or slightly longer) seems to kill the system completely, during that 10 second period, software may start to run and cause damage.

By far the preferred method is to remove power directly from the system by disconnecting it from the mains. Even this is not as straight forward as it may sound.

Instinctively, the correct way to do this would appear to be by switching power off at the wall socket and then removing the plug.

Unfortunately, doing this simple action may send a signal to the device that power has been lost and allow it to take action to damage potential evidence. This is because of the presence of an *Uninterruptible Power Supply* (UPS) (see Figure 3.1).

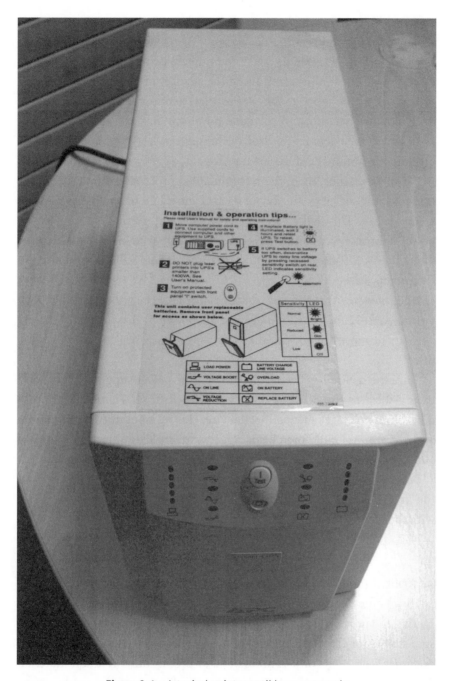

Figure 3.1 A typical uninterruptible power supply

A UPS is a battery which is kept charged from mains power and which is designed to supply power to a device even when mains power has been lost. Typically, it is used to allow servers and other systems to shut down cleanly when power is lost, thus minimising the chances of damage occurring. In order to allow the server to take appropriate action, the UPS has to be able to send it a signal informing it that a power-cut has occurred. This signal triggers software activity, in exactly the same way as pressing the power button, or running the shut-down process.

For these reasons, then, the recommended process is to pull the power lead from the socket on the device itself (Figure 3.2), or as close as possible to the device. This will ensure that there are no external UPS or similar power sources in circuit. Of course, there still remains the problem of internal power sources (e.g. laptop batteries). These will be considered in Chapter 8.

Note, however, that accepted practice is to allow any printing or CD/DVD writing to finish before disconnecting the power, as these produce a near-permanent record of activity that was happening when the machine was discovered.

Once the device has been isolated from the power supply, all leads and their associated sockets should be clearly labelled (see Figure 3.3), in case it becomes necessary to reconnect devices during laboratory examination, and everything should then be packaged and labelled to start the evidence audit/continuity trail (see Figures 3.4 and 3.5).

From this point on, whenever the device is handed over to any person, the label should be completed showing the date and time of handover along with the identity of the person it is passed to.

Additional items

During the process of acquiring the device itself, someone should take re-sponsibility for gathering associated documents such as notebooks, printed documents etc. that contain notes of passwords or other relevant material. The user or owner should also be questioned about passwords and encryption systems at this time.

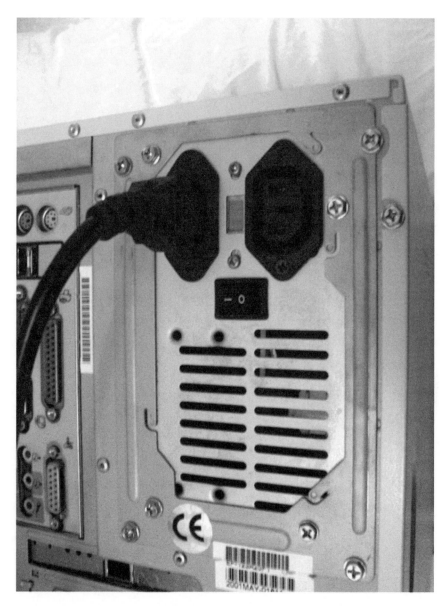

Figure 3.2 A standard power connector on the rear of a PC

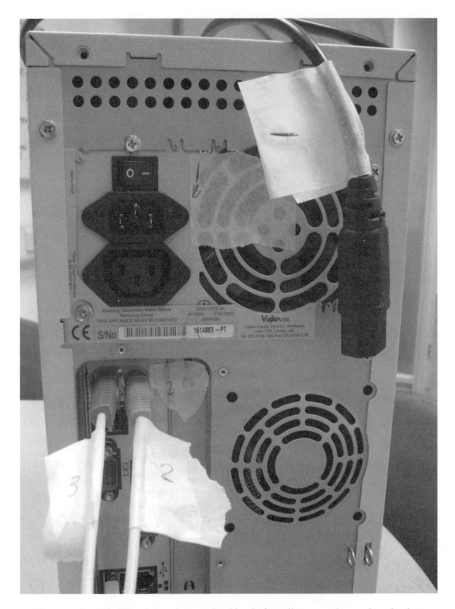

Figure 3.3 Labelling the sockets and cables before disconnecting and packaging

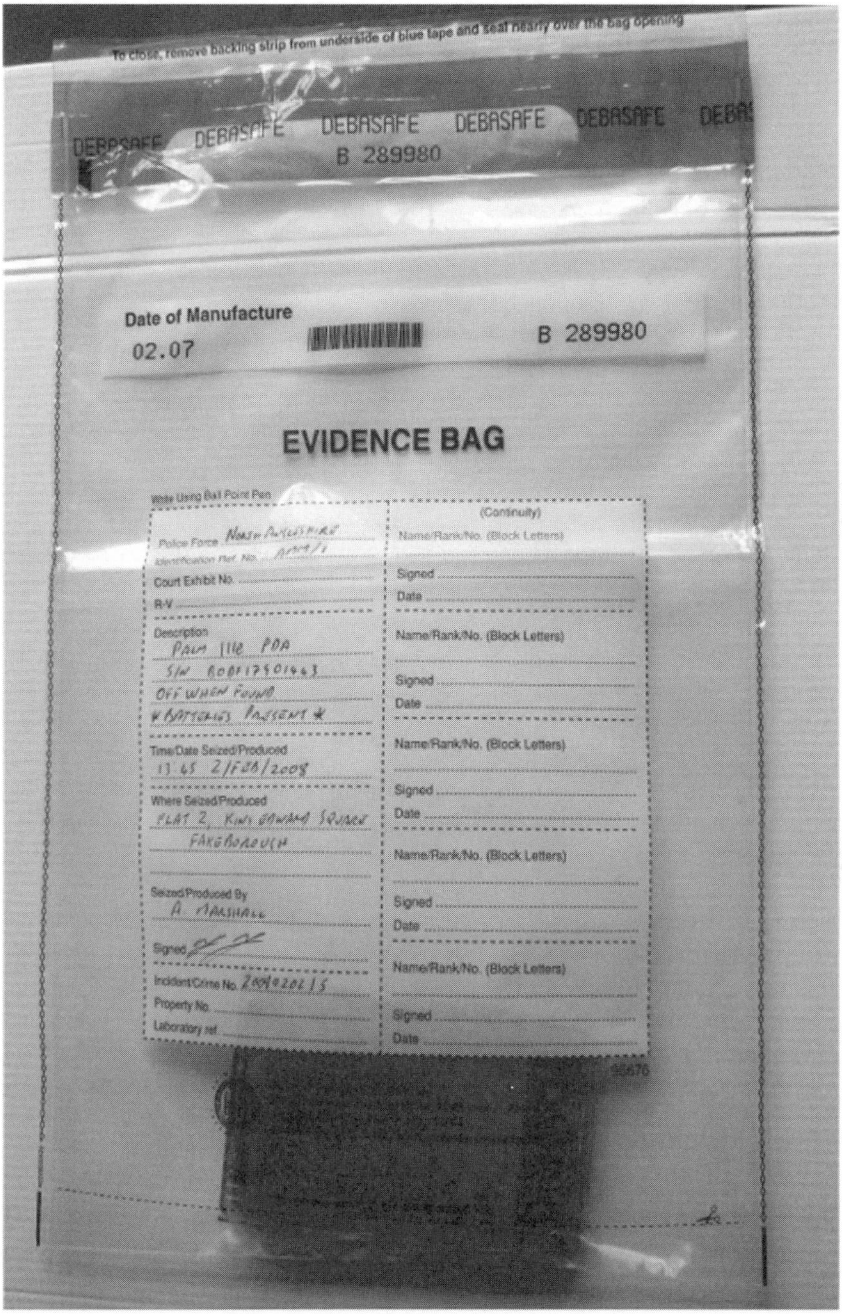

Figure 3.4 A PDA in tamper-evident packaging

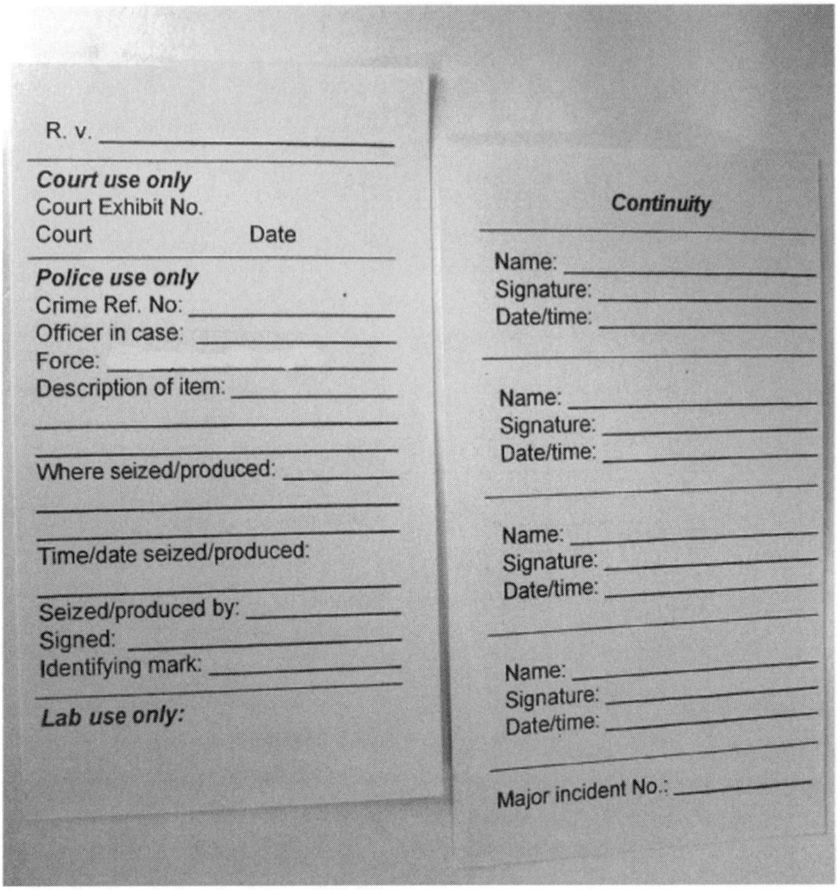

Figure 3.5 Front and rear of a sample evidence label, also know as a "CJA" (Criminal Justice Act) label

Threats and risks

Throughout the description of the seizure process, above, there has been constant mention of the fact that almost any interaction with a device being seized can cause changes to the state of that device. This is a real risk. If the state of the system, when it comes to be examined, can be shown to have changed during or after seizure, then the integrity of all data on that device can be challenged, effectively accusing someone involved in handling the device of tampering with it.

3.2 Device identification

From the discussion above, it may sound as if it is easy to identify digital devices. Most people have a very clear mental picture of a PC as a beige or black box with keyboard, mouse and monitor attached to it. Similarly mobile phones, media players etc. seem to be easily identifiable devices. However, the truth is that the onward march of Moore's law [32] (see Chapter 1) means that the "chips" at the heart of all devices are getting smaller and more powerful all the time. As a result, more features can be packed into smaller packages.

Combine this with the fact that digital devices have become lifestyle devices rather than purely technical solutions, and we have to incorporate the influences of design and fashion trends into any consideration of device identification.

3.2.1 Case modding

Amongst a certain group of owners, there is a fashion for case modification, aka "modding". Much as owners of mundane vehicles attempt to make them more attractive or unique by attaching spoilers, neon lights, chrome wheels and fancy paint schemes, case modders change the external appearance of their computers to make them more personal or attractive.

Web sites such as http://www.mini-itx.com/ (see Figure 3.6) contain details of readers' projects showing how they incorporate PCs into everything from whisky bottles to dolls based on Japanese manga characters.

As a result, PCs may no longer look like PCs, but can be disguised as household objects. Indeed, as the convergence between entertainment equipment and computing equipment moves forward with O/S such as Windows Media Center Edition allowing PCs to be used as video recorders and hi-fis, there is a desire to "improve" the appearance of computing equipment to make it fit better within the living environment.

Another approach taken to the problem of making computers more suitable for domestic use is that taken by manufacturers such as Shuttle

CVN-65 USS Enterprise Aircraft Carrier
By Russ Caslis - Posted on 21 January 2003

Introduction

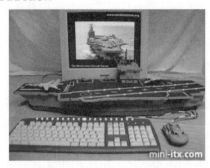

So I was walking around a toy store waiting for my wife to finish looking at the Barbie toys one day (before anyone asks, yes, she is more than eight years old and I love the fact that she is still into toys) and I saw this cool looking toy of the aircraft carrier Enterprise. I looked closer at it, and thought that it might be big enough to hold one of those great Mini-ITX motherboards from VIA. Since the toy was only $19.99, I decided to get it. Upon getting home, I ripped open the box and confirmed that the width of the toy at it's largest area was a little over 17cm wide. The Mini-ITX would be a tight fit, but it would work.

I could see it all now - runway lights, planes on the deck, control switches on the command center - it looked great. All that was left was the planning, cutting, building, painting, and tweaking. No problem!

In reality, it was a 4 month project that was more difficult than many would claim just by looking at the mod. Let's go over the individual pieces and show what it took to create the mod.

Mouse

At first, I bought a cheap ball mouse with the idea to paint it like a ship. I would have a "missile bay" on the back by placing rows of red/white/blue LEDs. I also masked off alternating sections of the white mouse cable and dyed the cable as well, leaving some sort of a warning tether.

Figure 3.6 Sample from `http://www.mini-itx.com/` showing a model aircraft carrier which contains a full PC (see Appendix A for more images)

and Apple, both of whom have produced "mini" computers which occupy little more space than a small stack of CDs and which are designed to look like ornaments or conventional small hi-fi equipment.

The only common factor with these devices is the need for them to have cables for power, video, network, keyboard and mouse. The last three of these requirements are disappearing, too, as wireless keyboards and mice become more reliable and wireless network speeds and reliability increase.

3.2.2 Novelty items

Another category of device which can pose problems is that of portable storage. Typically, these are lumped together under the catch-all terms

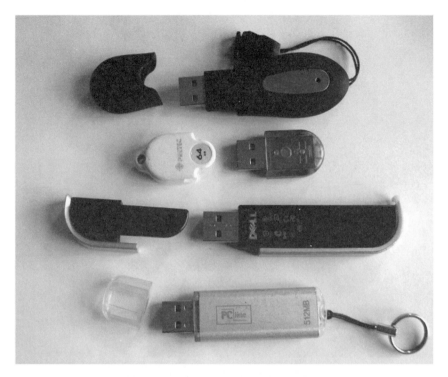

Figure 3.7   "Standard" USB storage devices

"thumb drives" or "USB sticks" because the earliest and most common versions of these USB devices were about the same size and shape as a thumb (see Figure 3.7).

Moore's law [32] plays a part here again. As the chips for these devices have shrunk in size and/or increased in capacity, the real limiting factor in their external design has become the USB connector itself. Outside of the requirement to have the right physical connector, there are no limits to the shape, size, colour etc. of these devices. Everything from wristwatches to toy dolls, via pens, fish-fingers, sushi and keyring footballs has been used as a casing for solid-state USB storage (see Figure 3.8).

3.2.3 "Purloined letters"

Although it is becoming easier to disguise devices through the production of customised cases, it is still easier to adopt Edgar Allan Poe's "purloined

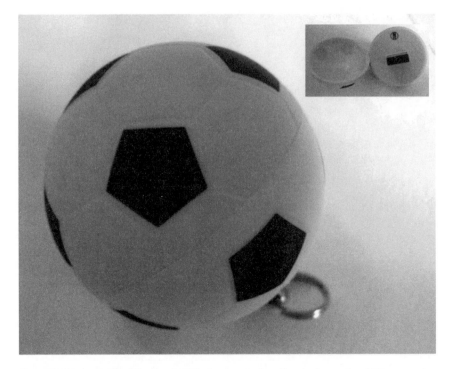

Figure 3.8 A novelty/disguised USB storage device (inset shows the USB connector visible when it is opened)

letter" [38] approach where the object is, effectively, hidden in plain view but disguised by being placed in such an obvious location as to appear not hidden, or is disguised as an inoccuous object.

As an example, consider a DVD on which a collection of illegal images of children (IIOC) has been written. The criminal may take steps to hide this under floorboards, behind a panel in the wall, or in some other secret location. Alternatively, he may choose to hide the DVD by simply placing it in a case for a commercially available DVD, possibly even going as far as printing a false label on it to further disguise its identity. If the illegal disc is then placed in a collection of innocent discs, its presence will be less obvious and more likely to be overlooked if a search of the disc collection is anything less than thorough.

This method has been employed to hide several different types of device and, with miniaturisation leading to devices such as micro-SD or Trans-Flash cards (see Figure 3.9) it has become possible to secrete large volumes

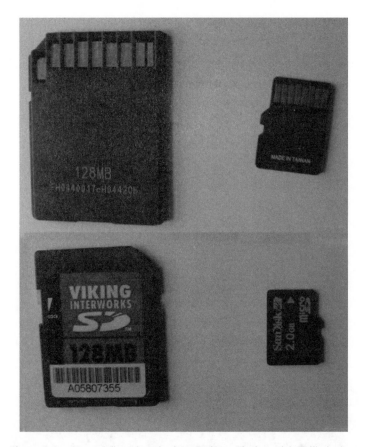

Figure 3.9   SD card (large) and micro-SD/TransFlash card (small) devices

of data in very small hiding places such as the spines of hardback books, children's coin banks and so on.

A further twist lies in the fact that storage devices can be shared by several other devices so that a single SD card (Figure 3.9) may contain photographs which are visible when it is used in a digital camera, but the same SD card may contain other images which are not accessible by the camera and only available when the card is used with a mobile phone or computer with card reader.

The underlying message, here, is that objects are not always what they appear to be and should be checked, thoroughly, to see if they may contain any digital devices. Equally, digital storage devices should not be assumed to contain only one type of data simply because of where they were found.

3.3 Networked devices

As mentioned earlier, networks can pose a particular problem during search and seizure. Apart from the threats mentioned above (Section 3.1.1), any form of communications immediately introduces the possibility that we are dealing with multiple machines. Where a wired network is present, it may be sufficient to trace the cables from the network socket (Figure 3.10) to the router (Figure 3.11) or hub/switch (Figure 3.12) used to connect the various machines together.

Cable tracing, though, may be complicated by the fact that cables can be run under carpets, below floors, through walls and through ceilings. Each time a cable passes through a wall, floor or ceiling its direction and point of exit may not be clear. Indeed, there may be a hidden hub, switch or router used to extend the network and split the connection to lead to even more machines. Irrespective of this, cable tracing should always be attempted. In this process, the presence of any of the devices mentioned can be helpful as the lights on the front of these devices give a good indication of which cables

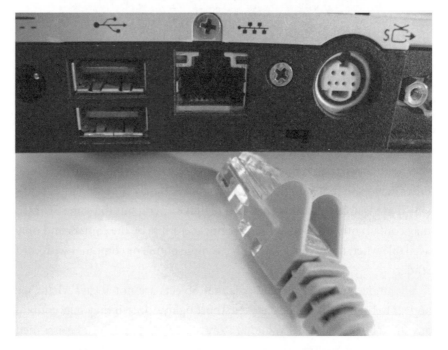

Figure 3.10   A network socket on a PC and associated cable

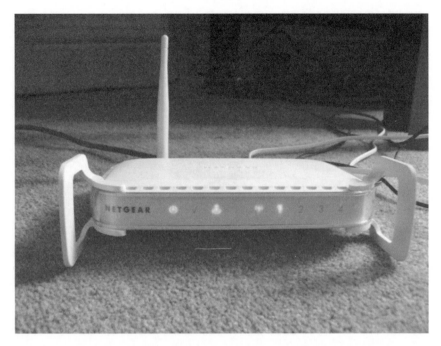

Figure 3.11 A domestic broadband router with wireless antenna

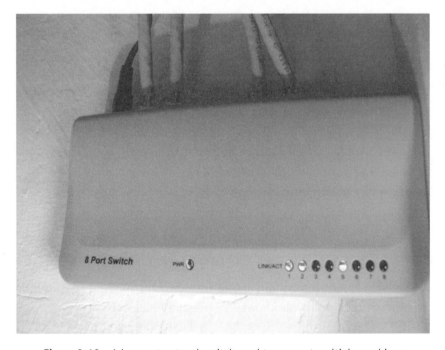

Figure 3.12 A low-cost network switch used to connect multiple machines

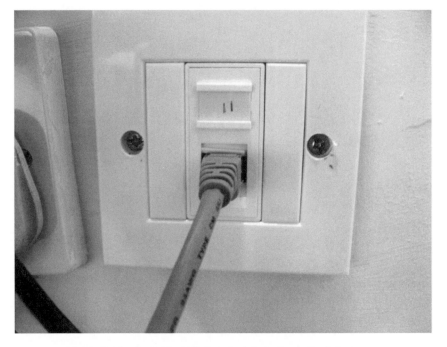

Figure 3.13 A standard RJ45 wall plate in the author's bedroom

are live and carrying data. If all cables have been disconnected from all but one obvious device,[2] but the switch is still showing data being transferred, there must be at least one more device attached to the network.

In the event that the network has been installed using standard RJ45 wall sockets (Figure 3.13), it is likely that all the wiring in the premises leads back to a central patch-panel (Figure 3.14) or switch (Figure 3.12) from which all live circuits can be located. This is most commonly found in business premises, but this method of network installation is becoming more popular in domestic situations.

3.3.1 Wireless

A relatively recent innovation is the introduction of the two common wireless network protocols known as WiFi and Bluetooth.

---

[2]Network traffic can only exist where two or more devices are connected to the network.

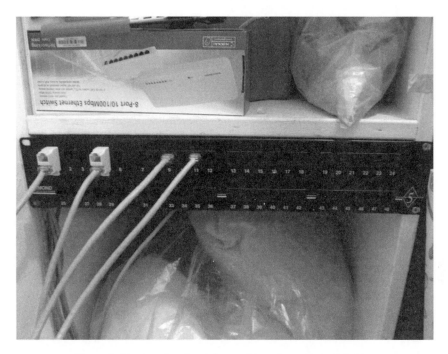

Figure 3.14 A network patch-panel in a domestic installation

The IEEE802.11 [23] family of wireless networking protocols for local area networks, often referred to as "WiFi", defines a set of standards using different carrier frequencies for medium to high speed networking over a limited range of 100 m (or more) in clear air (i.e. outdoors in ideal conditions). It offers similar features to wired networks, although speeds tend to be lower, without the requirement to physically plug-in to a network point. As such, it has become very popular in domestic settings as a way of sharing broadband connections without having to run cables to every room, and as an added service for travellers in cafés, coffee shops, hotels, airports and other places where it may be useful to use an ad-hoc network connection.

Bluetooth [6], meanwhile, offers a "personal" area network (PAN) designed to allow items of personal technology to work at short range (typically 1 m to 10 m, although the standard does allow for up to 100 m). The most popular use of Bluetooth, currently, is for hands-free headsets for mobile phones, although printers and various other devices are available in Bluetooth-enabled form.

If either of these technologies are in use in the vicinity of suspect equipment, it may be useful to know this. Since both are based on broadcast radio frequencies, it is possible to detect them using appropriate receiving equipment, such as a notebook/laptop computer equipped with an appropriate transceiver[3] card and specialist software which scans for the appropriate frequencies without attempting to connect to detected networks. Tools such as NetStumbler and Kismet have proved useful for the detection of IEEE802.11 networks, while BlueStumbler and similar tools perform the same function for Bluetooth systems.

3.3.2 Remote access

Whatever the type of network present, there exists the possibility that someone outside the premises has access to the equipment under investigation through the Internet. The ACPO Good Practice Guide [2] recommends that connections to the Internet should be disconnected immediately upon discovery.

Where no other advice is available, the ACPO recommendation is appropriate; however it should be remembered that a sudden disconnection from the network may alert remote users to the fact that the machines are under investigation. In an ideal world, monitoring of live Internet connections should be considered, although there is some debate about whether this constitutes wire-tapping or some other form of covert surveillance, with consequent concerns about admissibility of evidence gathered.

3.4 Contamination

In "conventional" forensic science, one of the major concerns associated with the handling and examination of any item of evidence is that of contamination or cross-contamination. The possibility of fibres accidentally being transferred between items, DNA mixtures appearing or fingerprints being deposited after an item has been seized have all caused problems when evidence has come to court in the past.

---

[3] Transceiver = transmitter/receiver.

In the field of digital evidence, similar concerns about contamination can arise and can be considered in two distinct areas: physical contamination and digital contamination.

3.4.1 Physical contamination

Although it is still not common practice for digital devices to be examined for physical evidence such as fingerprints, fibres and DNA, some work in this area [26] has suggested that physical evidence may have a role to play in corroborating or disproving theories about the physical processes undergone by devices. For example, examination of fingerprints and toolmarks on a hard disc may assist in determining if it has been replaced by the owner or if it is still the original installed at the factory. Consideration of the fibre population inside a PC may give some indication of whether it has been moved recently, and examination of fingerprints and earprints on a mobile phone may help to identify the most recent user.

For these reasons, care should be taken to ensure that opportunities for physical contamination are minimised during packaging, transport and laboratory examination of devices.

3.4.2 Digital contamination

Digital contamination is another serious issue. ACPO Principles 1 and 2 [2] require that steps must be taken to ensure that material held on storage devices is not modified in any way unless absolutely necessary. Unfortunately, the presence of wireless network equipment (see Section 3.3.1), with coverage that extends beyond the physical boundaries of the premises containing the equipment, presents new challenges.

It has become almost impossible to obtain notebook computers without WiFi [23] capabilities, or mobile phones without Bluetooth [6]. Technologies such as these present several opportunities for damage to digital evidence, either deliberately or accidentally.

A knowledgeable criminal may deliberately choose to use the technologies as "sniffers" constantly seeking new devices and, when a new device is detected, trigger software which destroys evidence held on the machine before it can be seized. Worse yet, a terrorist could use the same technique to count the number of unrecognised wireless devices within range and use this information to trigger an explosive device only when the threat to human life is maximised.

Another approach is to "pair" pieces of equipment using wireless methods. If one member of the pair is seized and taken out of range of the other (or even switched off), this can be treated as an unexpected event and, again, used as the trigger for some activity.

In all of these cases, the aim of the criminal is to gain advance notice of unwanted attention and to take steps to destroy incriminating material. The use of the wireless technology allows the process to be automated.

Another risk, though, arises from the possession of wireless-capable devices by those involved in investigating crime and seizing equipment. If care is not taken to ensure that the investigators' devices have had their wireless functions disabled prior to approaching a suspect device, there is the risk, not only that their devices will be detected as above, but also that their devices may carry out default behaviours to join local wireless networks. If the investigators' notebook computer, for example, is allowed to join the criminal's computer network, the state of machines on the network will change and ACPO Principle 1 will be violated. Similarly, a Bluetooth-enabled phone may attempt to pair with any other phone, headset or other Bluetooth device as soon as it detects its presence.

Ideally, then, no wireless-capable devices will be permitted anywhere that digital devices are thought to exist, unless they are in the hands of properly squalified personnel who have good reason to use them (e.g. in order to detect the presence of other wireless devices).

4

Examination Principles

As mentioned previously, the ACPO Good Practice Guide for Computer Based Electronic Evidence [2] requires that any examination of a digital device is done in such a way as to minimise the possibility of digital contamination. By implication, this means that all work should be carried out on a copy of the suspect device rather than the original and, in a perfect world, this would be the case.

There are circumstances, however, where it is not possible to seize equipment and produce a complete "forensically sound" copy. As noted in Section 3.1, we must ensure that any action taken is justified, appropriate and proportionate. In the case of a shared computer or network this can be difficult to achieve without performing some level of analysis at the time when the equipment is first discovered. This approach, often called *previewing* is also useful in the laboratory environment to assist in determining which devices should be given priority for examination due to the nature of their contents.

4.1 Previewing

The preview process may be considered to carry a significant risk of violating the ACPO's first principle, because it requires direct examination of the suspect devices. However, correct application of Principles 2, 3 and 4 provides some degree of protection from accusations of evidence-tampering.

Digital Forensics: Digital Evidence in Criminal Investigation   Angus M. Marshall
© 2008 John Wiley & Sons, Ltd

4.1.1 Offline preview

In a typical preview situation, the device to be previewed will be dealt with in an offline state. That is to say, it will have been disconnected from networks and shut down to allow the examiner to remove storage devices for connection to a trusted preview workstation. Ideally, devices will be connected through a write-blocking device to ensure that ACPO Principle 1 is still upheld.

This used to require specialist hardware for each device interface type in common use. A more modern approach, though, relies on the existence of the USB mass storage standard [50], which allows many different devices to be connected through the same standard USB interface. Because all these devices use the same protocol for communication, it is possible to use a common USB write-blocker (similar to that shown in Figure 4.1) to protect them against accidental digital contamination.

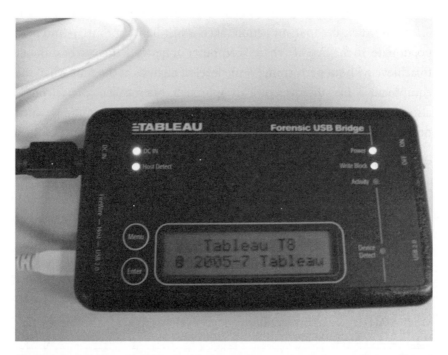

Figure 4.1 A Tableau T8 USB write-blocker used to protect devices against accidental data writing

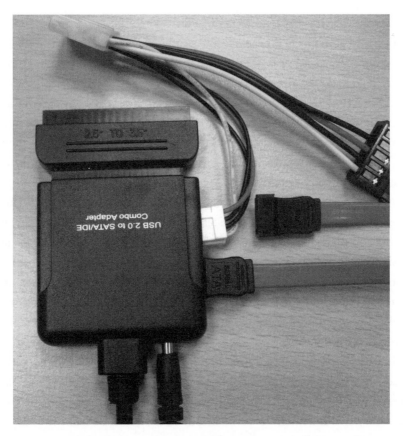

Figure 4.2 A typical SATA/IDE-to-USB hard disc adapter

The write-blocker is connected directly to the forensic workstation and the device under examination is then connected, possibly through an adapter such as that shown in Figure 4.2, to allow previewing to proceed.

Once the device has been correctly connected, previewing is conducted using software similar to that used in the laboratory, to gather information about the data held on the device and allow the examiner to judge the likely evidential value of the device as a whole.

4.1.2 Online preview

The benefit of offline previewing is the opportunity to use physical methods to prevent contamination of possible evidence. The major disadvantage with it, however, is the requirement to shut down the device under examination and gain physical access to the storage devices it contains.

In some situations, it is not possible to shut down the equipment and we need to consider an alternative approach: *online* previewing.

Conducting an online preview is, arguably, the most risky activity any digital evidence examiner can perform. By its very nature, the preview examination will be carried out on a live system, which is undergoing changes of state and which cannot be considered to be completely trustworthy.

Although some degree of previewing can be conducted using programs already present on the suspect system, it is difficult to show that they are giving complete and accurate results. Programs such as *rootkits*, which are designed to implant themselves into a system to allow an attacker to abuse that system, tend to contain features which alter system programs and functions to disguise the presence of the rootkit. Thus, any program which makes use of system functions must be considered to be inaccurate unless it can be proven otherwise.

In order to conduct an online preview, therefore, most examiners have access to trusted tools on read-only media such as CDs. These tools have been written in a trusted environment and the CD contains all the code necessary to allow them to run without using any code from the suspect system. They tend, also, to be written in such a way that they protect the suspect system from accidental changes to data, apart from the necessary changes to primary RAM[1] to run the trusted tools themselves. A list of useful tools and other resources can be found in Appendix B.

The aim of previewing is, generally, to establish something akin to "probable cause" in order to determine whether or not the equipment being previewed can legitimately be seized for laboratory-based examination. Although every attempt is made to follow the ACPO principles, it can be difficult to prove that the previewing process has not caused changes to data on the system and it may be difficult to use evidence acquired in this way for anything other than intelligence purposes.

---

[1] Random Access Memory – the memory used to run programs and store data while power is applied.

4.2 Imaging

As suggested above, the usual recommendation is that any forensic examination of a system should concentrate on storage devices, and that all work should be carried out on copies or images of those storage devices. This is similar to the requirements of the HOSDB Digital Imaging Procedure [11], which mandate that before any work is carried out on a digital photograph a write-protected *master copy* should be created and preserved and further *working* copies generated from it when necessary.

To produce an accurate copy of a digital storage device, we need to use a method which will produce a *complete* copy of the device, including all unused space, deleted data and, if possible, damaged areas. This is not a normal function of any standard software available to most users. Instead, specialist tools or standard tools with special options (see Appendix B) are used to get the most complete copy possible.

4.2.1 Offline

Offline imaging is the simplest procedure, although it can be time consuming depending on the size of the device to be imaged.

In this process, the suspect device is connected to an imaging workstation using a write-blocker, as described in Section 4.1.1. The imaging software is then used to read data from the device and store it to either a file or separate device. Once imaging is complete, the first copy is usually considered to be the master copy and further working copies can be generated as required. Of course, there is still a requirement to show that the master copy and working copies are completely accurate and have not been modified in any way during imaging or examination. Mechanisms for dealing with this issue are discussed in Section 4.3.

4.2.2 Online

When it is not possible to seize or shut down the suspect system, or where the storage device is difficult to connect to the imaging workstation, it may be necessary to use online imaging. In this situation, the storage device is left *in situ* and live imaging tools are used to capture data from it using the accompanying hardware. Of course, this poses similar problems to online previewing, but the use of trusted tools goes some way to mitigating these. The trusted tools allow the examiner to copy the device to either an external storage device, such as a USB hard disc, or across a network to a dedicated storage server.

4.2.3 Backups

One final method can be used to collect data from a suspect system and is particularly applicable in business environments. Backup tapes or discs produced over a period of time can allow the examiner to build up "snapshots" of system states at the time backups were produced. Although these will contain only files which were live and scheduled for backup, the material contained in them has proven useful in the past. It must be remembered, though, that any image produced from backups is only a partial image and that hidden data is unlikely to be found in this situation unless multiple backups can be used to produce images of the system at various points in time.

4.3 Continuity and hashing

Once an image of a storage device has been created, the image and the device need to be treated as if they were crime scenes, with all that means for preservation of evidence and avoidance of contamination and tampering. In the physical world, this is achieved by establishing cordons/quarantine zones and ensuring that all activities are subject to thorough recording.

The use of write-blocking methods should ensure that original devices are not subject to modification, but additional checks can be used to demonstrate that the processes used by the examiner have had no adverse effects on either original or image. These methods can also be used to alert the examiner to any accidental changes, allowing him/her to check and re-check processes which seem to be problematic.

Table 4.1 Hash values for strings which differ by one bit

String	Computed MD5 Hash (in Hexadecimal)
12345678	23cdc18507b52418db7740cbb5543e54
12345679	0f4fd7804fbbcf67df5dc8ef8dc946fb
22345678	0c7e888e4e214b74c1ec2b6734096fe6

Hashing algorithms similar to checksums are used to calculate digital "signatures" which are effectively unique for any piece of digital data. At the highest level, one or more hash values will be computed for the data on the original device. Because the image has been produced from this device, and contains identical data, the hash value for the image should match, exactly, the value for the original. Hashing algoriths such as MD5 [42], SHA-1 [36] and SNEFRU [31] are very sensitive to changes in data, and the modification of even a single bit (1/8 of a byte) in the largest image results in radically different hash values being calculated (see Table 4.1 for an example).

Some tools use hash values for sub-elements of an image to allow the location of any modification to be found more easily, and provide additional assurance of evidence integrity.

Good tools also provide comprehensive logging facilities, allowing them to produce a complete list of all actions performed on the evidence during examination, helping to fulfil the requirements of ACPO Principle 3 [2].

4.4 Evidence locations

In examining any device to recover and analyse material present, there are four primary types of file or data which the examiner will typically consider. These can be summarised as:

1. Live data

2. Deleted data

3. Swap space

4. Slack space.

4.4.1 Live data

Live data are the data present on a system in a format which makes them accessible to the user or the normal software directly. Typically, they represent the outcome of some normal operation of the device or software as a result of deliberate action.

Generally speaking, live data have greater evidential value as they can be shown to be directly related to something the user of the system has chosen to do. Furthermore, because live data files are created and managed by the operating system on behalf of the application software, they tend to have reliable timestamps, insofar as the device's clock can be trusted.

Timestamps

Most operating systems maintain three timestamps for each file on the system, known as the *MAC* (Modified, Accessed, Created) times:

1. Modified: this records the time that the file was last modified, i.e. when it was last saved.

2. Accessed: records when the file was last read. On many operating systems this only records the date of reading, not the time on that date.

3. Created: records when the file first appeared on the system as a new file.

These timestamps are just one area of file *meta-data* which can prove useful in determing the sequence of events and nature of activity on a system.

4.4.2 Deleted data

Following on from live data, perhaps the next most useful area to consider is the deleted data on the system. This represents material which was live at some point in the past, but which the user or operating system has chosen to remove from the system for some reason.

Fortunately for the forensic examiner, most operating systems do not completely erase deleted data. Instead, they typically mark the area of the storage device occupied by those data as available for re-use. This is done because, historically, deleting data was a large, time-consuming task and it was (and still is) far easier to simply mark space as available for re-use and overwrite it when necessary.

The disadvantage of this, for the criminal, is that there is a good probability that old data can be recovered using appropriate tools. Unfortunately, because the files have been marked as deleted, their meta-data can no longer be considered entirely reliable, so information such as the MAC times cannot be relied upon in the same way as it is for live data.

4.4.3 Swap space

Another common feature of modern operating systems and applications is the ability to use storage devices as if they were part of the machine's primary RAM. Historically, and today, this has been done to make a machine appear to have more main memory than is physically present, as a way of keeping the cost of hardware down. Real primary RAM costs, on average, about 10 times as much as disc storage.

The method is similar to that of dealing with a phone call whilst in the middle of attempting to solve a difficult problem. As soon as the phone starts to ring, signalling that a new task is about to begin, the smart thing to do is to write down information about the problem and thoughts so far. Once the phone call has been dealt with, ideas can be reloaded into the brain by reading the notes made before the phone was answered.

The swapping process is completely automated and under the control of software. The user can usually only choose how much disc space can be used as swap space, but cannot choose which programs or pieces of data will be swapped out and in.

As more data and programs occupy main memory, the system monitors memory usage and identifies those areas which are least used in terms of frequency of use, recency of use or some other measure. When main memory becomes too "crowded" to accomodate new software or data, the operating system chooses which parts of memory to store to the disc and re-allocate for new data or programs.

Later, when the program which originally owned the memory needs access to it again, the operating system chooses a new area to swap out, stores this to disc and then loads the original data back into main memory.

Since the user has no control of the process, it is possible to find data in swap space which has never been written to storage devices for any other reason. Swap space is often a good source of information about passwords for encrypted files and other sensitive data.

Because swap space is in constant use, and has no particular meta-data associated with it, it is difficult to determine exactly when data were deposited within it.

4.4.4 Slack space

Finally, we can consider slack space: data which are stored alongside live data, but not deliberately put there by the user.

Slack space tends to arise because of some properties of storage devices and filesystems which dictate that there is a minimum quantity of data which must be written to, or read from, a storage device. The exact size of this *Minimum Allocation Unit* or *MAU* varies from filesystem to filesystem. The larger the MAU, the greater the chance that slack space may contain useful data.

Figure 4.3 shows how the use of MAUs leads to slack space being created when data are written to the sorage device. If the program requesting the write provides insufficient data, the system is free to grab data from anywhere in memory and use it to pad the data to be written to ensure that the MAU is completely filled. Again, the user has no control over how the system chooses which areas of memory to use as padding.

In this case (Figure 4.3), three blocks are completely filled, but there is slack at the end of Block 4, which must be filled with other data from some location in RAM.

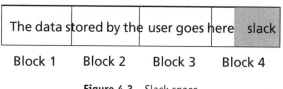

Figure 4.3 Slack space

Because data in slack space are written at the same time as the real contents of the file, the modified time in particular can be used to show that the data were present in main memory at the time the file was written. The data in slack space are not made available to programs as a result of file reading, so the accessed time has little or no significance in this situation.

5

Evidence Creation

Any piece of data or software in a digital system may be evidence, if it has some meaning relevant to the investigation. In order to determine which software or data we need to consider, it is useful to think in terms of how these came to be present on the system we are examining.

We have already considered, in Chapter 4, *where* the examiner may find material on a system, but now we are starting to consider *how* it arrived on the system in the first place, and what it might mean as a result.

To understand something about this, it must be remembered that digital devices exist only to perform actions on behalf of their users. Although they contain many automated functions, all of their activity is performed as a result of instructions by a human being at some stage, and they exist only to process data as an aid to human activity.

Some security specialists argue that the involvement of a digital device in a crime represents a failure of the security surrounding that device. Since devices are concerned with information storage and processing, it is said that the information security has failed in some way and, although this viewpoint may be valid, it does not always tell the whole story. Some crimes can be committed without breaching any information security, but simply by using devices in the correct way for apparently proper purposes. The fault lies outside the system itself and relates to how it can be used to facilitate activites involving other systems and people.

One approach that can help to understand where evidence may be entering the system uses a seven-element model of information security [47]

Digital Forensics: Digital Evidence in Criminal Investigation   Angus M. Marshall
© 2008 John Wiley & Sons, Ltd

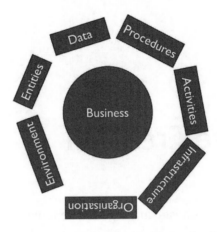

Figure 5.1   A seven-element model of information security

(Figure 5.1). Although the model does not directly show how anything may have arrived on a system, it does allow us to consider the elements, both digital and non-digital, which comprise the whole system, and thus allows us to consider how it has been used and what it has been processing. If we understand something about how it may have been used in committing the crime, we can direct our investigative resources most appropriately.

5.1 A seven-element security model

This model is based on a holistic approach to security, acknowledging that security depends on all elements of the system being secure in their own right, and showing the inter-relationships between key parts of the system. It contains seven key elements which are inter-linked to compose the system as a whole. Each of these elements must be secure in its own right and depends on its neighbouring elements to ensure this. If there is a weakness in any one of the elements, the whole system is insecure and may be attacked/abused through the weak element(s).

5.1.1 Entities

Entities are objects which can manipulate and/or be manipulated by the system, and may be passive or active. Passive entities are, generally speaking, external to the system, and are represented by collections of data which the system processes in some way. Active entities tend to be part of the system and are responsible for choosing and controlling which processing should be performed. Entities can be people, organisations or other types of object.

In security terms, we need to consider the behaviours of active entities and ensure that they are only allowed to behave in inherently secure ways. We also need to think about how changes to the system affect entities and whether those changes have been properly assessed for risk. Finally, the inter-relationships between entities may lead to insecurity through inappropriate interactions or through inferences being drawn about unknown entities based on information provided about known entities.

From an investigative point of view, entities are generally either the users of the system, some of whom may be involved in the unwanted activity, or they are potential targets of the unwanted activity because they have some value to the criminal.

5.1.2 Environment

In this context, the environment represents the set of constraints or restrictions imposed on entities in an attempt to make them behave correctly. Depending on the entities under consideration, the environment may be defined in terms of: legislation, ethics and regulation; technical capabilities and resource limitations; compatibility with other entities, interaction standards and procedures; or physical limitations. Examination of the constraints and restrictions contained in the environment may allow us to quickly identify any unconsidered vectors of abuse present in the system and, indeed, determine if it is feasible to proceed with an investigation.

In some circumstances the environment may prevent us carrying out an investigation because the activities required would break some of the laws which make up that environment. Equally, if we cannot identify applicable laws, policies or rules which prohibit the activity under consideration then, no matter how thorough the investigation is, there can be no action taken against the perpetrators. We can, of course, take action to ensure that the unwanted activity does not happen again.

5.1.3 Organisation

While the environment represents the complete collection of restraints and controls, the organisation contains the framework which allows those restraints and controls to be created, enforced and inter-related to each other while still allowing entities to co-operate and collaborate as necessary.

If the organisation is inadequate, then any investigation will struggle for lack of support, co-operation and resources.

5.1.4 Infrastructure

Infrastructure is the supporting mechanism required to enable activities within the organisation. It is generally composed of physical components (such as buildings, power supplies, computers, network switches etc.) which do not need to be considered as entities, but rather as enabling hardware. In some environments, the infrastructure may be more nebulous, for example the trading floor of a stock exchange would be an infrastructure, but it still has its own security requirements which act to protect the elements identified.

When considering an investigation, the infrastructure, or some part of it, is the crime scene that will contain the information we are seeking. In order to be able to identify the limits of the scene, we must have access to an adequate "map" of the infrastructure, showing how it is structured, in order that we can attempt to identify the boundaries of the critical components.

5.1.5 Activities

Activities are complete tasks, often representing a complete transaction, from end to end. Activities can be single procedures (see Section 5.1.6), but may be composites made up of multiple procedures.

Insecure activities are those which are poorly defined or understood and which have the potential to allow unwanted side-effects to occur. A good understanding of the activities in progress during the incident being considered should allow the investigator to reconstruct the sequence of events which led up to the incident, taking account of unexpected behaviours.

5.1.6 Procedures

At the procedure level, we are considering single tasks which represent discrete, identifiable, atomic (indivisible) processes within the wider context of an activity.

For example, making a cup of tea is an activity, with a clearly defined start and end point, which is made up of procedures such as "putting water in the kettle", "putting tea in the pot" and so on.

Procedures should be the smallest steps involved in an activity which may be shared with other activities (e.g. "putting water in the kettle" is shared with "making a cup of coffee").

Really, here, we are applying classical top-down design methodology to understand more about the actions taken within the system. By breaking them down into procedures which can be described simply and quickly, we increase the chances of identifying any that are weakly defined or more likely to result in unwanted or unexpected results.

5.1.7 Data

Finally, we come to data: the representation of the entities which the system is concerned with manipulating. Two key areas of security apply to data. Firstly, the system must have a mechanism to ensure that data integrity is maintained, i.e. there must be a way to make sure that all data held are accurate and can be maintained correctly. Secondly, the data must be protected from accidental damage or leakage.

In most environments, these goals can be achieved by ensuring that adequate backups are maintained (including ensuring that backups are restorable) and that data are protected from prying eyes through mechanisms such as strong encryption or physical restrictions placed on the storage devices.

Because data represents something about entities, such as details of bank accounts, it is often seen as the direct target of an attack. Any failings in data security, through flawed procedures, activities, infrastructure, organisation, environment or entities, leaves the system vulnerable.

5.1.8 Application to investigation

By mapping any system onto this seven-element model, it is possible to discover where the weaknesses in the system lie, and hence possible to identify which parts of the system allowed the unwanted activity to occur. It does not, however, always allow us to identify exactly how that activity took place. For this, another model which considers the possible interactions with the system is useful.

5.2 A developmental model of digital systems

In "Silicon pathology" [28] it is proposed that a digital system has a pattern of development similar to the growth and education of a human being. It is also suggested that, in this context, there are four particular routes by which any data or program can arrive on a system. These are summarised in Table 5.1.

This model suggests that any system can be used by two different classes of user – *Authorised* and *Unauthorised*. Put simply, authorised users are those who have been granted permission to use the system at the time

Table 5.1 Routes by which data/programs can arrive on a system

	Knowing Act	*Unknowing Act*
Authorised	Authorised user deliberately installs (*AK*)	Authorised user accidentally installs (*AU*)
Unauthorised	Unauthorised user deliberately installs (*UK*)	Unauthorised user accidentally installs (*UU*)

under consideration, leaving everyone else in the category of unauthorised users.

Although it may seem strange to include consideration of the time of usage in the definition of an authorised user, it can be significant. When we examine a system to discover how it has been used, often the only clue to who might have used it is the presence of confirmation that a particular user identity has been used to log in to the system. If it is not possible, or usual, for the legitimate owner of that user ID to be active at the time in question, further enquiries are necessary to determine if the user was that person, or some other person who has acquired the user ID tokens for some reason. Thus, even though we may have an accurate record of a user ID becoming active on a system, no responsible digital evidence examiner should ever report this as confirmation that that particular person was responsible for the activity. At best they will state something similar to "the activity was associated with the user account".

Misuse of a user ID does not necessarily indicate malicious intent. In spite of attempts to educate users and enforce correct user ID and password usage controls, in line with good information security [46] policies, it is all too common for users to share IDs and passwords in order to make life easier for each other.

This may have something to do with the perceived value of identity tokens such as user IDs and passwords [29], but a full exploration of this is beyond the scope of this book.

Whatever the reasons for insecurity of ID tokens, it is a fact of life that systems and identities can and will be shared.

It is also a fact of life that users can and do make mistakes, leading to the two types of activity (or vectors) defined in the model – *Knowing* and *Unknowing*.

5.3 Knowing

Vectors classified as knowing define any activity where the user is aware of the consequences of their actions. For example, a user who chooses to install a new word processor, having first spent some time investigating the changes that such an installation will make to their system, would be classified as a knowing act.

This category extends to cover situations where a user chooses to install software or create data using software from a trusted source, relying on the integrity of that source to ensure that there are no adverse or unwanted effects.

However, the knowing category also includes deliberate acts intended to implant illicit software or data on a system, providing the person responsible has made a conscious decision to abuse the system in this way. This implantation may be done for any one of many reasons.

5.3.1 Consumption of illegal material

A user may choose to deliberately download material which breaks the law in any way, ranging from copyright violation to illegality of content (e.g. illegal images of children). Because the act of downloading requires several deliberate acts: finding the download site, selecting the file(s), and selecting the file names under which to save them, the actions can be declared to be knowing. The user in this situation may be either Authorised or Unauthorised and determination of this status can be crucial to successful prosecution.

5.3.2 Implantation of illegal material

Following on from deliberate consumption, we turn to deliberate implantation of illegal/illicit material. Again, the motives for performing this act are varied and can range from simple revenge/extortion through to deliberate abuse of someone else's system to turn it into a distribution node, thus masking the origins of the material and allowing criminals to operate more freely by granting a degree of anonymity. In this instance, it is likely that the user will fall into the Unauthorised category and is likely to be operating covertly at the very least. However, if steps are not taken to thoroughly examine the system for the possibility of Unauthorised Knowing acts of implantation, prosecution may be difficult.

5.3.3 Zombies and Bots

Taking the concept of implanting material on someone else's system for the purpose of distribution leads us to the final example of knowing acts – those of Zombies and Bots.

In network security terms a Zombie is usually defined as a computer which has had software installed upon it, allowing a third party to take partial or complete control of that system without the user's permission or intervention. A Bot, meanwhile, is a system which contains software which can give the impression of autonomous operation. Zombie Bots can, and do, exist.

Zombies have been used in the past to set up large networks of compromised machines in order to launch co-ordinated attacks against web servers and other systems. Bots, on the other hand, are routinely used to harvest e-mail addresses, send spam,[1] illegally copy web material, acquire credit card numbers, impersonate human beings in chat rooms and many other acts.

The knowing category makes no distinction between the intentions of the person carrying out the installation, mainly because the examination of a storage device which has been subject to data/software deposition probably contains no information whatsoever about the state of mind of the person responsible at the time of the events.

5.4 Unknowing

The case of unknowing installation of software/data deals with the situation where the person apparently responsible could not have reasonably been expected to know or predict that their actions were about to cause damage.

This category deals with situations where a user is attempting to perform one action but, because the tools they are using are flawed or have been compromised, their actions permit some unwanted activity to occur.

---

[1] Spam = unsolicited commercial e-mail.

5.4.1 Web-site effects

In the author's experience as an expert witness for both prosecution and defence dealing with cases involving images of child abuse, one of the most common questions asked has been "could the images have been placed there as a result of a virus or pop-ups on a web page?". The questioner is really asking whether there is any indication that the images arrived as a result of a knowing or unknowing act, given that the person who was using the machine is already known to be an authorised user.

In the case of web pages it is very easy, by using the HTML "<img=...>" tag amongst other methods [28], to cause a web browser to download images which cannot be seen by the user. In legitimate sites, this technique is used to get images onto the user's machine so that they are available when the user clicks through to view other pages.

Alternatively, the web site may have been designed to open pop-up or pop-under windows, which appear over or below the desired page, respectively. Typically, this method is used in order to force an advertisement to appear on the user's screen.

Both of these methods allow a third party, the web site manager/designer, to cause material to be downloaded to the user's computer when the user chooses to view particular pages on their site. The user usually has no advance indication that the page they are about to view contains any of the code necessary to cause any of the actions mentioned above.

In these cases, the user is responsible for activity which falls into the *AU* category, while the person who created the webpages is responsible for *UK* category activity.

5.4.2 Stowaways

Another possibility is that a user has chosen to install a piece of software, or download a batch of files such as music in MP3 format.

To most users, these actions present no obvious risks, but it is perfectly possible that downloaded files may contain more than they appear to. The act of downloading is a category *AK* activity and this can be demonstrated by the fact that the user must give a location and/or name for the file(s) to be downloaded to. Their interaction with the dialog box which prompts them to provide this information gives them a chance to cancel the download. By giving the information and clicking on "Next", "OK", or "Proceed" they have given evidence of their consent to the download proceeding, strongly suggesting that thay have deliberately chosen to accept that material onto their computer. However, where they are downloading something like a .ZIP archive file, which is a container for many files, they have no way of knowing the exact contents of that file until it has been fully downloaded and uncompressed. If the creator of the compressed file has chosen to include additional files, some or all of which are illegal in nature, then the user has apparently downloaded those files at the same time as the ones they really wanted. The act of downloading is classified as AK, the package creator's act is also AK, but the user's possession of the illegal files can be defined as AU.

5.4.3 File sharing

Consideration of file downloading, as above, leads naturally to the issue of file sharing. Programs such as Limewire, eMule, Kazaa, BitTorrent and Gnutella are designed to allow many users to share complete or partial files to allow them to be transferred more quickly around the community. The software itself has many legitimate purposes, but is also regularly used for illegal distribution of material.

Most file sharing systems are geared up so that the user must choose which files they wish to either download from, or make available to, the rest of the community of users of that particular file-sharing network. Once a file has been downloaded, in full or in part, the default is to make it available to all other users, thus increasing the efficiency of the whole network. Popular files are available from more places. Files obtained from these networks are subject to the same caveats as for any other downloaded file. The person acquiring the file can, almost certainly, have no guarantee that the contents are "as described" until the whole file has arrived.

Some systems, however, operate more like the file sharing found in operating systems. They allow the user to share a folder or part of their storage either as read-only or read/write storage with other users on the network. If the storage area is shared as read/write it is, of course, possible for other users on the network to place files onto it without the owner's knowledge. Although the external users appear to be authorised, whether all of them actually are authorised remains open to debate, as does the issue of which parties are knowing and unknowing . . .

5.4.4 Malware

A final area to consider in this section is that of Malware. Malware is simply defined as softWARE with a MALicious purpose. Typically it comprises the family of programs known as Viruses, Worms and Trojan Horses.

A *virus*, in the digital world, is any program which is capable of replicating itself from one system to another, through some carrier medium, without direct human action. Its propagation is, therefore, *UK* facilitated by *AK* because an unknown and unauthorised person deliberately created it, but the action of an authorised person may be required to enable its distribution. In the 1980s, viruses were transferred mainly through the use of floppy discs being swapped between machines. As in the biological world, a virus cannot exist without a host, so viral software spread by infecting other programs, effectively becoming a stowaway within legitimate programs.

In 1988 Robert Morris accidentally created the first Internet *Worm* [45]. Morris's intention had been to write a program which could calculate the size of the Internet. His aim was to create a program which would hop from machine to machine by exploiting flaws in the security in certain key programs. His design was too successful and contained a serious flaw.

If the worm was only going to explore the Internet, once it had catalogued each machine it should have reported its findings, infected a new system and then died, returning the infected machine to a "clean" state. Morris's worm did not always do this. In approximately one in seven cases, the worm became immortal and continued to send out infections to other machines on the net. Machines which had previously been infected became re-infected, increasing the chances that they would acquire an immortal version of the worm. The net effect was that within a very few hours, a huge number of machines had been subjected to the attack and the Internet itself was suffering from a "traffic jam" caused by all the worms seeking out more machines to infect.

This attack is clearly of type *UK* – an unauthorised user has knowingly created a piece of software which places itself onto other systems. However, it could be argued that there is also a *UU* component to it, as the severity of the attack goes beyond the original intention.

Modern worms follow this type of behaviour, exploiting new security flaws, in order to plant sofware onto infected machines. Often this software may not cause another machine to be infected, although many do, but may instead plant another program which serves the purposes of a remote criminal.

Finally, we have the group of malware known as *Trojan Horses*. These are programs which arrive, carried with or by some other program (worms or viruses), and which implant themselves in the system to cause further damage, allow a remote attacker to take control of the machine in order to acquire information from it, or to turn it into a distribution node for e-mail spam, web pages, images or any other files. In these cases, Trojan Horses are now commonly spread through viruses or worms, via infected systems. This mechanism provides the criminal with added security as an investigation needs to trace the origin of the material back to the infected machine and from there back, possibly through a long chain of infected machines, to the originating system. By the time the origin is discovered, it is likely that the criminal will have moved on and have become effectively untraceable.

Since malware has the potential to infect any machine, a responsible examiner should always check for the presence of malware or artefacts indicating prior infection, and report their findings. Most of the major anti-virus software firms maintain databases of malware which describe, in some detail, the effects of each virus, worm or Trojan Horse detected.

It must be remembered, though, that anti-virus software tends to operate in the same way as the human immune system. Action to eliminate the invader is only taken after infection has taken place. Anti-malware software can only be created after the malware has been detected and analysed. There will always be a period of time during which successful malware can spread freely.

5.5 Audit and logs

Implicit in the discussions above is the assumption that sufficient information about the system exists to allow the models to be applied. Correctly
specified systems will have been subject to rigorous specification and testing
prior to deployment, and there will be audited records of everything that
has officially happened to them in their lifetimes. Unfortunately, in all but
the largest organisations, this process tends to be avoided or done badly.

More realistically, the investigator will be dependent on the recollections
of the owner/administrator/user about what they think they have done,
coupled with any information that the system may have recorded in its own
og files. Some systems record copious amounts of data as they are running,
and this can be an invaluable starting point, but others are incapable of
recording anything because of the way they are designed or because of
limitations on storage space available.

For these reasons, it can be vital for a full audit of a system to be conducted
early in an investigation in order to attempt to identify the installed elements
and compare with lists of known good or bad components. Time-line
analysis, based on the MAC times present is also useful in aiding attempts
to identify when system modifications occurred.

6
Evidence Interpretation

Once the means by which unwanted data (which includes software) have arrived has been identified we can start to consider its meaning. To achieve a thorough consideration of this we need to think about what the data actually are (*Data Content*) and where they are (*Data Context*). As discussed in Chapter 5, it is possible for illicit material to arrive as a result of innocent (*Unknowing*) actions and, although the material is clearly evidence of a crime, the person responsible for it arriving on a system may not be deliberately or directly involved in the criminal act itself.

6.1 Data content

Data content is, as the name suggests, concerned with the meaning of the data itself. It deals with interpretation of stored data, based on the contents of files.

6.1.1 Data meanings

The starting point for any examination of data content must be the determination of how data can be interpreted. At heart, all digital files consist purely of binary (1s and 0s) data which can be read in many ways (see Table 6.1 for examples). As standard, binary digits (*bits*) are read in groups of 8 (8 bits = 1 byte), 16 (word), 32 (double word) or 64 (quad word). The

Digital Forensics: Digital Evidence in Criminal Investigation Angus M. Marshall
© 2008 John Wiley & Sons, Ltd

Table 6.1 Possible meanings of some byte-length binary strings

Binary String	One's Complement	Two's Complement	Unsigned	Binary Coded Decimal (BCD)	ASCII	EBCDIC
00000001	1	1	1	1	Start of Header	Start of Header
00010001	17	17	17	11	Transmit On	Transmit On
01000000	64	64	64	40	@	Space
01000001	65	65	65	41	A	No-break Space
10000000	−0	−127	128	80	*no meaning*	*undefined*
10000001	−1	−126	129	81	*no meaning*	a

standard used is determined, first of all, by how the processor in the machine accesses memory, but secondly by how software chooses to represent data.

From the processor's perspective, binary data may be program instructions, addresses of data in memory, or just raw data used by programs. This meaning may not become fully clear until the processor starts to work with the data, and the meaning may change at different points in the processing.

Programs usually base their internal data processing on one of the many data encoding standards already defined, but are free to use any representation which their programmers choose to create. For example, an older word processor may use 8-bit data interpreted as ASCII[1] or EBCDIC[2] to represent the text it works with. These character representations can be quite limiting as they contain little allowance, if any, for the use of different alphabets in different parts of the world. A more modern word processor would use 16-bit UniCode [49] to allow mixed-alphabet documents to be used.

Without any indication of the intended meaning of a binary string, it can be read in more than a dozen ways – each of which is equally likely to be correct.

6.1.2 File extensions, signatures and magic numbers

Because data files can, and are, shared by different programs, mechanisms for passing information about file content have been developed. For the user, extensions to the filename are commonly used, with well-known

---

[1] American Standard Code for Information Interchange.
[2] Extended Binary Coded Decimal Interchange Code.

Table 6.2 Sample file signature "magic numbers"

File Type	Binary Preamble	ASCII Signature
Microsoft Cabinet (.CAB) file for software installation		MSCF
Microsoft XBox (.XBE) program		XBEH
Portable Network Graphics (.PNG) file	01011001	PNG
JFIF JPEG (.JPG) file	11111111 01101000	JFIF
MPEG2 layer 3 (.MP3) audio file	11111111 11111010	

(If a column is blank, there is no data in this format in the header.)

abbreviations such as ".DOC", ".JPG" and ".PDF" being used to help human beings identify files of similar type.

For software, however, the filename has little or no meaning. Instead, most programs use a sequence of bytes at the beginning of each file to determine the nature of the data held in the rest of the file. These file signatures, also known as "magic numbers" are defined for most file types and can be found in reference tables available online (see Table 6.2 for a few examples). The signatures are not all the same length and may begin several bytes into the file, using a mixture of raw binary and otherwise encoded data to identify the true purpose of the file.

Many files also have a defined footer or trailer which is used to identify the end of the file and may have special meaning to programs which understand that type of file.

Ideally, an examination will use complete files with intact headers and footers, but in extreme circumstances it is sometimes possible to "guesstimate" the original type of file which contained an unattached fragment of data, based on its contents alone. This can be difficult to justify and explain, but does have uses where files have been partially overwritten.

6.1.3 Compression

Many data representations are considered to be inefficient and wasteful of space or network bandwidth. Something like English text, for example,

Table 6.3 The alphabet in Morse Code

A	. −	B	− . . .
C	− . − .	D	− . .
E	.	F	. . − .
G	− − .	H	. . . .
I	. .	J	. − − −
K	− . −	L	. − . .
M	− −	N	− .
O	− − −	P	. − − .
Q	− − . −	R	. − .
S	. . .	T	−
U	. . −	V	. . . −
W	. − −	X	− . . −
Y	− . − −	Z	− − . .

contains many repetitions and, in ASCII, EBCDIC or UniCode, uses the same number of bits to represent common and uncommon letters alike. In the days when telegraphy was a major communications method, this problem was known and Samuel Morse's code (Table 6.3) used shorter patterns of "dots" and "dashes" for common letters to allow operators to transmit messages more quickly. Other innovators developed Morse's principles further by using special codes to represent whole words. In the modern world, we have seen a resurgence of this method in the appearance of "txt-spk" (text-speak, Figure 6.1) where abbreviations and altered codings are used to represent common phonemes and words in mobile-phone short messages.

All of these methods share a common purpose: they aim to reduce storage space or transmission time by changing the representation of the data without destroying any of the information carried.

Lossless compression

Lossless compression desribes a family of mechanisms by which data can be transformed into smaller representations without losing meaning. Detail

Txt	English
TY C.U. l8r.	Thank You. See you later
lol. soz. g2g. txt bck.	Laugh Out Loud. Sorry got to go. Text back

Figure 6.1 Examples of txt-spk

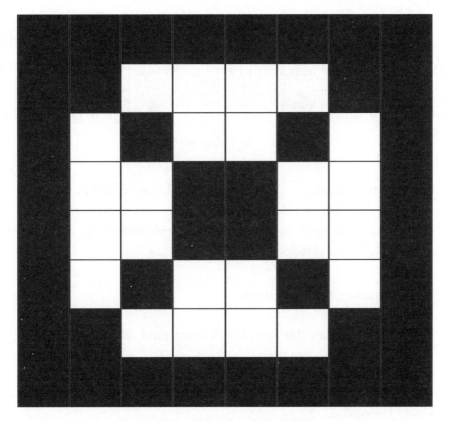

Figure 6.2   Image to be compressed

of some of these mechanisms is beyond the scope of this book, but the principle can be demonstrated with some simple examples.

Consider the picture shown in Figure 6.2. This is a 10×10 grid in which each pixel (picture element) is either black or white.

Representing this image using the simplest method entails recording every pixel exactly as it appears. For this image we can use one byte value to represent black (giving it the value 11111111) and one byte value to represent white (00000000). Figure 6.3 shows the picture as a 10×10 grid of bytes (i.e. it requires a full 100 bytes to represent the whole picture).

Inspection of this binary representation reveals that it is made up of only two bit patterns and that we could make significant savings if we could reduce the number of bits required to represent each pixel. Because there are only two colours, it would make sense to use a single bit to represent

11111111	11111111	11111111	11111111	11111111	11111111	11111111	11111111	11111111	11111111
11111111	11111111	00000000	00000000	00000000	00000000	00000000	00000000	11111111	11111111
11111111	00000000	11111111	00000000	00000000	00000000	00000000	11111111	00000000	11111111
11111111	00000000	00000000	11111111	00000000	00000000	11111111	00000000	00000000	11111111
11111111	00000000	00000000	00000000	11111111	11111111	00000000	00000000	00000000	11111111
11111111	00000000	00000000	00000000	11111111	11111111	00000000	00000000	00000000	11111111
11111111	00000000	00000000	11111111	00000000	00000000	11111111	00000000	00000000	11111111
11111111	00000000	11111111	00000000	00000000	00000000	00000000	11111111	00000000	11111111
11111111	11111111	00000000	00000000	00000000	00000000	00000000	00000000	11111111	11111111
11111111	11111111	11111111	11111111	11111111	11111111	11111111	11111111	11111111	11111111

Figure 6.3   "Raw" image in binary form

either white (0) or black (1), but in order for this mechanism to work for an arbitrary number of colours and allow accurate reconstruction of the original image, we need to introduce a colour table into the file. So, we can define a file header as follows:

- byte 1 number of colours present

- byte 2 colour code 1 (bit pattern used to represent colour 1)

- byte 3 colour value 1 (original colour in the image)

- byte 4 colour code 2

- byte 5 colour value 2 . . .

The length of the bit patterns used in the image will be determined by the number of colours present so, in our case, although we are defining the bit patterns in bytes, only the right hand side (least significant) bit will actually be used as we only required a single bit for two colours. Applying this, our 10×10 grid becomes that shown in Figure 6.4 and occupies just 100 bits which is just $12\frac{1}{2}$ bytes.

Even with the addition of the file header, which contains the details of the original colours in the image and the bit patterns used to represent them, the compressed file is still only $17\frac{1}{2}$ bytes in length, considerably smaller than the original, but without losing any of the original information.

Of course, the example given above is a little artificial and does not work for all images, but it adheres to the main principle of lossless compression:

1	1	1	1	1	1	1	1	1	1
1	1	0	0	0	0	0	0	1	1
1	0	1	0	0	0	0	1	0	1
1	0	0	1	0	0	1	0	0	1
1	0	0	0	1	1	0	0	0	1
1	0	0	0	1	1	0	0	0	1
1	0	0	1	0	0	1	0	0	1
1	0	1	0	0	0	0	1	0	1
1	1	0	0	0	0	0	0	1	1
1	1	1	1	1	1	1	1	1	1

Figure 6.4 Compressed image using one bit per pixel

no information has been destroyed. Its representation has just been transformed into something more efficient.

Compression of this type is particularly appropriate where damage to the original information cannot be tolerated, and can be applied to files such as word processor documents, databases, spreadsheets and financial records.

Depending on the nature of the data to be compressed, a range of more advanced lossless compression techniques may be used and the reader is advised to look at Lempel-Ziv (LZ) [53] and Huffman [22] as good starting points if more detail is required.

Lossy compression

Lossy compression takes compression a stage further, accepting that not all information is always required. In photographs, video and audio in particular there is often much detail which goes unnoticed by the human eye, or which is imperceptible to the ear. If these "unnecessary" components can be identified and discarded, an acceptable impression of the original is retained, but in a much smaller file which can be further compressed using lossless techniques.

When the file's contents need to be reproduced, the software will interpolate, filling in the missing detail based on the information remaining in the file.

For most purposes, this results in an acceptable representation of the original in spite of the loss of information. However, if the compression

Figure 6.5   Original uncompressed image: file size 320 kilobytes

algorithm is forced to attempt too high a level of compression, too much information will be deleted and the decompression software will be unable to produce a good replica of the original. Figures 6.5 6.6 and 6.7 show JPEG images with varying levels of compression. Figure 6.7, in particular, shows how badly images can be degraded by over-compression using lossy methods.

As the images show, the loss of detail between Figures 6.5 and 6.6 does not significantly impact our perception of the overall image, although careful inspection shows some loss of detail in the buildings and water. Figure 6.7, on the other hand, is unrecognisable, showing unacceptable degradation.

Historically, this has been a source of debate about the admissibility and use of compressed digital photographs for forensic purposes, but it is now accepted [11] that, except in situations where any detail loss is unacceptable, they provide an adequate representation of the object being photographed and can be used in the same way as conventional "wet film" photographs.

Figure 6.6   Image compressed using JFIF JPEG set at 50 per cent quality: file size 24 kilobytes

6.1.4 Composite files

In the early days of computing, application programs tended to work with only one type of data and required only simple data files which contained all the information appropriate for the task in hand. These monolitihic files provided only simple storage capabilities, but were adequate for their intended purpose and many applications are still capable of working with those simple files.

However, as we have moved towards more mixed or multi-media applications, files have become more complex to the point where modern data files used by word processors, presentation programs, spreadsheets etc. may have to hold a mixture of numerical, textual, graphical and audio data all at the same time. These "composite" files typically exist in two forms: *Segmented* and *Compressed Folder*.

A segmented file appears, superficially, to be a monolithic file, but is usually a sequence of data "chunks", each one containing a different part

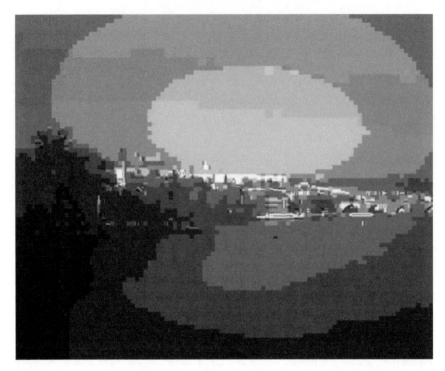

Figure 6.7   Image compressed using JFIF JPEG set at 10 per cent quality: occupies 4 kilobytes

of the data required for the document in question (see Figure 6.8 for an example). This allows a single file to contain different media types in a manner which allows all the individual elements of the document to be kept together for storage and transfer.

More recently, though, programmers have started to explore the possibilites of XML [51], the eXtensible Markup Language, as a way of producing

Segment Number	Content
1	Table listing other segments
2	Definitions of styles for paragraphs, characters etc.
3	Document text containing reference to embedded images etc.
4	Image 1
5	Image 2

Figure 6.8   An idealised sample segmented file structure for a word-processed document

catalogues of the elements which need to be combined to produce a document. They have created an expanding family of *composite* files, such as the Open Document [37] and DOCX [15] standards, which mainly consist of a compressed directory or folder holding all of the document elements. Within the directory, the document elements are held as individual files, along with a XML "manifest" file detailing the nature and purpose of each of the files in the directory.

The net effect is similar to that achieved by the segmented file, but modification to the composite file can be made more easily, as each component can be edited individually. Moreover, because of the use of XML, there is potential for new features to be added in a way which does not prevent older versions of the programs from handling newer files correctly.

6.1.5 Encryption

The use and even the very existence of encryption technology has provoked much debate and controversy over the years. There are those who believe that it should have no place in a civilised society and that no-one should be permitted to use it, while others accept that it offers an essential means of protecting privacy and freedom of speech. Whatever your point of view may be, the reality is that strong encryption systems exist and are freely available to anyone who cares to buy or download them. As a result, some criminals choose to use encryption in an attempt to disguise their activities.

Under the terms of the Regulation of Investigatory Powers Act [21],[3] usually shortened to RIPA, failure to disclose encryption keys is an offence punishable by up to two years in prison. Obviously, if the offence under investigation carries a longer sentence it may be preferable, from a criminal's perspective, to be found guilty of the RIPA offence whilst preventing any evidence of a more serious offence being uncovered.

The goal of any encryption system is to scramble the original data or message in such a way that no unauthorised person can decrypt it to recover the original content. This is usually done by ensuring that only authorised

---

[3] And its equivalent in Scotland.

Plain Text	A	B	C	D	E	F	G	H	I	J	K	L	M
Cipher Text	M	N	O	P	Q	R	S	T	U	V	W	X	Y
Plain Text	N	O	P	Q	R	S	T	U	V	W	X	Y	Z
Cipher Text	Z	A	B	C	D	E	F	G	H	I	J	K	L

Figure 6.9 A simple shift-substitution or "Caesar" cipher table

recipients have access to the encryption "key". This key takes many forms: it may consist of knowledge of the actual encryption method use; it may be a secret word, phrase or number needed to decode the data; or it may even be some physical feature of the recipient (such as a fingerprint) which can be used to generate a unique key for that person.

Over the years, encryption has developed a long way from the simple subsitution cipher [44] (see Figures 6.9 and 6.10), often credited to Julius Caesar, where each letter of the alphabet is replaced by a single other letter, thus obscuring the message's contents to the casual observer.

Simple ciphers, such as the Caesar cipher, are susceptible to easy decipher-ing using statistical cryptanalysis methods based on knowledge of the lan-guage thought to have been used to construct the original message. In our example (Figure 6.10), the letter "E" appears most often, as it does in written English, and we could deduce that it has been subsituted by "Q" in the ci-phertext. This leads us to the key that A becomes M, B becomes N and so on.

If the key is not quite as obvious, we could perform further analysis based on knowledge of letter frequencies in written English and deduce each letter used in the message individually. Couple this with our knowledge of how words are spelt, and a few minutes of effort would break this cipher easily.

More complex ciphers aim to break the patterns present in the data by using more complex keys and manipulating data at lower levels. Typically, a modern encryption system will use a key of at least 1024 to 2048 bits as the basis for its encryption. By combining this key with the original binary data, the resulting encrypted data can appear to be nothing more than random gibberish. However, the very randomness of the resulting file can at least assist us in detecting the presence of encryption through an "entropy" test.

Plain Text	Cipher Text
THIS IS AN ENCRYPTED MESSAGE	FTUE UE MZ QZODKBFQP YQEEMSQ

Figure 6.10 Application of the cipher table in Figure 6.9

Files with high entropy appear to be highly random and, as noted above, this is often a good indicator that encryption has been applied. If we can determine the software used and obtain the key, possibly using the methods described in Chapter 4, then the encrypted data can be recovered.

If we are unlucky, though, it may be necessary to attempt a "brute force" decryption attack where many different algorithms and keys are tried until the data are recovered. The complexity of modern encryption means that such attacks may take several months or even years to complete successfully, if at all.

6.1.6 Steganography

An alternative, or adjunct, to encryption is the use of steganography, or data hiding, to disguise the presence of material. This concept, too, predates the computer age, and its existence can be traced back for several centuries. Allegedly, one of the early examples of steganography involved shaving a man's head and then tattooing a map on it. Once the hair had grown back, the existence of the map was hidden from sight and only those who knew it was there would seek out the carrier.

In more recent times, secret agents have reduced photographs to the size of a full stop on this page and stuck them on pages of text. Again, only someone who knows where to look is likely to find information hidden in this way.

The content of a file may, itself, contain hidden meaning. For example, a terrorist leader who releases a video clip to television news channels may have arranged various "props" in the background and the presence and positioning of those props may communicate a message. The ordering of items in a shopping list, choice of music or desktop wallpaper may also be used in this way.

However, for our purposes, we shall concentrate on digital steganography. Modern steganographic methods rely on properties of files to allow data to be combined to produce an innocuous carried file which contains the secret information. As outlined in the earlier parts of this chapter, digital files have specific structures and may, as a result, have areas which are under-used or amenable to modification without significantly affecting their use.

Most current research on steganography is concerned with methods for embedding, and detection of embedded content, in files produced through lossy compression. Because these files are already distorted representations of the original, it is possible to make minor modifications to them without affecting the user's perception of the reconstructed image, movie or sound. As an example, consider a single pixel in a photograph. Effectively, within the file, information is stored about the colour present in each pixel. This may be as an absolute colour value, typically using eight bits for each of Red, Green and Blue (giving an RGB triple) where 00000000 00000000 00000000 is pure black, 11111111 00000000 00000000 is Red and so on, to 11111111 11111111 11111111 giving pure white. Alternatively, it may be stored as a value which represents the colour of that pixel relative to those around it (e.g. one unit "bluer", three units "red-greener" etc.).

No matter what the representation used in the file is, the ultimate goal is to allow it to store something like the original information in a way which the user perceives as "good enough". Making changes in the low-order bits (i.e. those which have least impact on the resulting value) does change the reconstructed image, but in a manner which is almost imperceptible (00000000 00000000 00100010 is not a very different shade of Blue to 00000000 00000001 00100010). Thus a single byte of hidden content can be distributed across several pixels, making a very small change in each.

So, the human being will not perceive the changes, particularly if they do not have access to the original information, but appropriate software which knows the embedding mechanism can extract the hidden data on demand.

Detection of this type of embedding, currently, tends to rely on either knowing the signatures of common embedding programs (i.e. common patterns which always seem to appear where these tools have been used), or statistical analyses of files which measure deviation from the normal profile of known "clean" files.

Other possibilites exist in segmented and composite files. It is entirely possible that additional data can be added to these files, but since it is not used by the reading program, it will be invisible to the regular user. In this case, detection can be performed by careful inspection of the segment table or the manifest and identifying those parts of the file which are clearly unused in the carrier document.

Even when steganographic content can be detected, though, it is often found to be encrypted . . .

6.2 Data context

While there is little doubt that, in terms of initial evidence, file/data content is crucial, all that it really provides is evidence of the existence of those data on the device being interrogated. In order to determine something more about how the data arrived and what they mean, we need to consider the context in which they exist.

As previously discussed in Chapters 4 and 5, every file on a system should have timestamps associated with it, detailing when the file was created, last modified and last accessed. Consideration of these timestamps allows us to build up a picture of the sequence of events during a period of usage. The closer that period of usage is to the time of seizure, the more accurate or complete the sequence of events will be.

Also of significance is the exact name and location of the file within the filesystem.

By default, many programs automatically create data files in special areas of the filesystems which are, effectively, reserved for their use. Usually, these "reserved" areas will be located in common areas which the user would not normally be expected to explore.[4]

Files found in these areas, therefore, tend to indicate that a particular progam was in use at the times indicated by the files, but may indicate nothing more than an automatic action of the software.

Files found in other areas, however, such as the "My Documents" folder tree in Windows, tend to have stronger evidential value. For a file to appear in these areas, or for it to have a name which is obviously meaningful to a human being, tends to indicate that the user has made a conscious decision to create and manipulate that file, with that name in that location. As mentioned in Chapter 4, this meta-data is not necessarily preserved when the file is deleted, but it will always exist for live files.

---

[4]Most of these reserved areas can still be inspected and manipulated by a knowledgeable user.

Thus it is possible to have lengthy discussions and debate about not only the nature of data content, based on how different programs may interpret the data, but also on the meaning of the meta-data and the significance of a file found in one location as opposed to a copy of it found in another. This issue will be explored further in Chapter 7.

7

Internet Activity

Although the categories of device involvement in crime (Chapter 2) distinguish between closed and open systems, it is now a reality that the vast majority of digital devices lie within the open category. Either they have (or have had) a direct connection to the Internet, or have been connected to some Internet-connected system at some point in their lives. As a result, analysing and interpreting evidence of Internet activity has become a crucial part of the investigator's role.

To understand something about how the Internet works and leads to evidential opportunities, we need to know something about networks in general.

7.1 A little bit of history

Relatively early in the short history of computing, it was realised that it would be useful to allow machines to exchange information without having to resort to "sneakernet"[1] as the primary communications method.

The earliest attempts to allow this relied on the use of modems and telephone lines to allow direct communication between machines, on demand. However, this type of network was soon recognised as inefficient,

---

[1] An academic network technique involving the use of PhD students wearing sneakers to transport data disks from one machine to another.

Digital Forensics: Digital Evidence in Criminal Investigation   Angus M. Marshall
© 2008 John Wiley & Sons, Ltd

particularly when three or more machines needed to communicate at the same time.

Some of the most important work led to the development of the ISO/OSI seven-layer model of networking [24]. Although this network has rarely been directly implemented, it is a useful model to consider as it allows us to explore the functions of various parts of networking technology independently. The main structure of this model has been in-corporated into today's most popular networking system – the Internet Protocol.

7.2 The ISO/OSI model

The ISO/OSI model divides the functions of a network into seven layers based on the services each layer provides and requires (see Figure 7.1).

Each of the seven layers is concerned with a single key function and provides a service to the layer above, while using the services provided by the layer below. The great benefit of this type of model is that the network can adapt to embrace new technologies by fitting them into the appropriate layer(s). If done correctly, there is little or no impact on the layers above or below and software can exploit the new functions with no modifications at all.

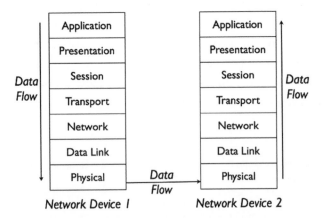

Figure 7.1   The ISO/OSI seven-layer network model

7.2.1 Application layer

The application layer is the highest level in the network stack and represents the languages used by programs to communicate with each other. The protocols in this layer tend to represent discrete actions required by the software to support specific operations and, on the whole, are designed to support client-server model activities where one program (the client) requests a service of the other (the server). Some systems operate in a pure client-server model, where it is obvious which component is the server as it completely controls access to its resources. Others, however, operate more like peer-to-peer systems, where all programs provide both client and server functionality.

A client-server system is sometimes described as "fast-food computing". In order for a customer (client) to get access to the food, they must issue a request to the shop assistant (server) who will fetch it for them, or make them wait until it is available. If the server is busy, the clients have to queue and await their turn.

7.2.2 Presentation layer

The presentation layer defines the network equivalent of the alphabet to be used for communications. That is to say, it defines the individual language elements which are used to represent the application layer protocol. This layer can be responsible for translating between different character sets (e.g. ASCII to EBCDIC and back again) and may also be responsible for implementing the encryption used to provide secure communications across an untrusted network.

7.2.3 Session layer

Moving down the stack we next encounter the session layer which is responsible for maintaining a dialogue between two pieces of software. This layer is the lowest one at which we can distinctly identify individual conversations. The session layer separates traffic passed to it by the transport layer and ensures that the various fragments of "conversation" are sent to the correct recipient. As an analogy, it can be thought of as the person who delivers letters to the correct offices from a central mailroom that receives all post for the building. It has a particularly important role at the beginning and end of any dialogue as this layer is responsible for ensuring that the communications session is established and closed correctly.

7.2.4 Transport layer

While the session layer is concerned with program-to-program communications, the transport layer deals with end-node to end-node (or source machine to destination machine) communications, and is responsible for combining multiple sessions into a format suitable for transmission between machines, making best use of the available communications bandwidth.

To do this, the transport layer typically breaks up session-layer data into chunks, known as "packets" which can travel independently of each other. At the receiving end, the corresponding transport layer gathers packets together and re-assembles the data contained in them into something which can be passed to the session layer.

It is a little like a courier travelling from one building to another. All the letters produced by the session layer are handed to the courier and delivered to the correct building. At that building, the transport layer (courier) hands the letters over to the session layer (mailroom) for delivery to the correct office.

This layer can usually detect simple communications failure and deal with non-receipt of data by requesting re-transmission from the corresponding transport layer at the other end of the communications channel.

7.2.5 Network layer

The network layer is the route planner of the stack. Its concern lies with identifying the most efficient way of getting the transport layer's data from point of origin to destination. This may involve pre-planning a route and attaching information about it to the data before it is sent, or it may involve individual intermediate nodes making their own decisions about the best route on a case-by-case basis as each chunk of data is processed.

Although the transport layer views the connection between two machines as a continuous channel full of packets, the network layer may implement it as a series of "hops", passing data from one machine to another until the final destination is reached. The exact route taken by each packet may change based on network conditions, or it may be the same for all, depending on how the network layer has been told to behave.

The network layer also attempts to monitor the state of those parts of the network that it uses, and adjust its routing tables appropriately to suit prevailing conditions, unless instructed to use static routes for certain communications.

7.2.6 Data link layer

Sitting between the network layer and the physical layer is the data link layer. It is responsible for implementing the network hops used by the network layer, and deals with adjacent node-to-node communications. As such, it is aware of the real structure of the network as created by the physical implementation, and often uses a different type of address to identify a particular piece of hardware. Since this address is the one used on the communications medium and which, effectively, controls access to the data link layer, it is usually known as the *Medium Access Control* address. For most devices, this address is set at the point of manufacture and is not normally changed without very good reason.

The data link layer also repackages data from the network layer into chunks (or frames) which are more suitable for transmission by the physical layer.

7.2.7 Physical layer

At this lowest level of the network stack, the data link layer frames are converted into something which can be transported through the medium which carries the network. This can be electrical impulses for wired networks, light for optical networks or radio frequency signals for wireless networks.

7.3 The Internet Protocol suite

The development of the Internet Protocol (IP) suite, in the late 1960s and 1970s is possibly one of the most significant events in human history. Until this point, all networks tended to be tied into particular manufacturers and hardware, but the IP suite, with its layered model, created a de-facto standard which everyone could, and did, adopt. A large part of the popularity of this technology also comes from the fact that all significant developments have been subjected to public discussion, scrutiny and publication through the RFC (Request For Comments) mechanism adopted in the early days of its development. Through this system, anyone was free to propose a new standard for internetworking and subject it to inspection by the rest of the community. This, in a manner similar to the development of modern open-source software, led to the creation of robust standards which could be implemented by all.

Nowadays, the RFC mechanism is still used, although in a more formalised manner, and RFCs are archived online in various locations such as `http://www.rfc.net/` and `http://www.rfcs.org/`.

Where the ISO/OSI model proposes seven layers, the IP suite contains only five (see Figure 7.2), merging or distributing some of the ISO/OSI functions within those layers.

7.3.1 Application layer

In the IP suite, the application layer combines the functions of the application and presentation layers in the ISO/OSI model. At this level we find protocols such as HTTP (the HyperText Transfer Protocol used in most common WWW applications), SMTP (Simple Mail Transfer Protocol), POP-3 (Post Office Protocol 3), FTP (File Transfer Protocol) and all the

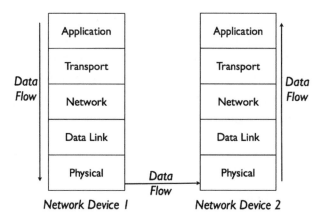

Figure 7.2   The IP suite five-layer model

others regularly used by individual pieces of software. Some of these are discussed in more detail later in this chapter.

7.3.2 Transport layer

IP's Transport layer shares some of the functions of the session and transport layers in the seven-layer model. Two main protocols are used at this level: the Universal Datagram Protocol (UDP) and the Transmission Control Protocol (TCP).

UDP, sometimes also known as the Unreliable Data Protocol, places emphasis on rapid delivery of data from one point to another, but gives no guarantee that all data will arrive as intended. It is particularly useful for applications where large quantities of data need to be moved quickly, but where quality of service is not a particular issue. Typically, streaming audio or video services, such as Internet radio or TV, will use UDP as the occasional hiccup in sound or pictures can be tolerated.

TCP, on the other hand, includes mechanisms for guaranteeing that lost packets will be re-transmitted once their loss has been detected. Therefore, although it can provide no particular guarantee about speed of delivery, it is favoured for applications where there needs to be a guarantee that all data will be received completely and correctly.

In both these protocols, the source and target applications at each end are identified by unique *port* numbers. Each protocol has 65536 ports available and they are probably easiest to understand if thought of as extension numbers in a telephone system. Calling the central switchboard ensures that the right company has been reached, asking the operator for a particular extension makes sure that the session is then handled by the right person or department.

7.3.3 Internet layer

The internet layer is broadly equivalent to the network layer of the ISO/OSI model, providing network management and routing services. It is in this layer that we encounter the legendary "*IP address*" which every machine on the Internet needs in order to be able to send and/or receive data.

At the time of writing, the vast majority of IP addresses in use are from the original IPv4 system, although most operating systems now support longer IPv6 addresses, which were introduced to deal with the impending shortage of unique addresses and allow for greater expansion of the Internet. At heart, both addressing systems use similar mechanisms to assist traffic routing, so we will concentrate on IPv4 as the simpler of the two to describe.

A standard IPv4 address is actually a single 32 bit number but, for ease of use, is usually written as a sequence of 4 bytes, known as a "dotted quad", as in 127.0.0.1. Historically, three main blocks of IP addresses were available for public use, allocated as:

- Class A networks beginning with 0.x.y.z to 127.x.y.z (i.e. 0.0.0.0 to 127. 255.255.255). Effectively this class consisted of 128 large networks, with the network identified by the first byte, and the machine within that network by the remaining three bytes.

- Class B networks beginning 128.0.y.z to 191.255.y.z (i.e. 128.0.0.0 to 191.255.255.255). These networks were smaller than Class A and identified by the first two bytes, with the remaining two being used to identify the node within the network.

- Class C networks beginning 192.0.0.z to 223.255.255.z (i.e. 192.0.0.0 to 223.255.255.255). In these networks, only 255 nodes are available (from the last byte) with the leading three bytes being used to identify the network.

Within these networks, three special networks were reserved for experimental or internal use and their addresses should never appear on the public Internet. These are the networks beginning 10.x.y.z, 172.16.y.z and 192.168.0.z to 192.168.255.z. Several other blocks of addresses are reserved for other purposes, inculding the 127.x.y.z network which always represents a virtual (non-physical) network that exists inside each and every Internet-capable machine.

The use of one part of the address as a network identifier, with the remainder as the node identifier, simplifies the job of delivering data from one place to another by splitting the delivery task into two stages. The first stage uses the network prefix to deliver data to the correct network; once this has been accomplished, the receiving network can use the rest of the address to ensure that data is sent to the right node.

Address allocation under the "classful" scheme shown above is recognised to be wasteful, so most modern networks now use a modified system called CIDR (Classless InterDomain Routing) addressing to allow any number of bits to be used for network identification with the remainder of the 32 used for node identification. Under this system, addresses are usually written as a dotted quad followed by the number of bits used for the network ID (e.g. 172.16.8.33/12 means that the first 12 bits are the network address and the remaining 20 are the node address).

7.3.4 Data link layer

This is the equivalent of the seven-layer version's data link layer, and is still responsible for node-to-node communications as directed by the Internet layer. The exact detail of this depends on the underlying physical layer but for most Internet systems there will be either a MAC address, associated with a network card, or a telephone number associated with the physical communications channel. Somewhere in the network there will be a record of the relationship between IP address and data link layer identity. However, it should be noted that, since IP addresses can be allocated on demand and thus systems may have different IP addresses at different times, it is vital to know the exact time that an IP address was in use if it is to be traced accurately.

7.3.5 Physical layer

Finally, the physical layer continues to convert data link layer frames into appropriate signals for the transmission medium.

7.4 DNS

Although, at machine level, the Internet relies on the use of IP addresses, these are less than intuitive and not particularly useful for most humans.

To solve this problem, a system to allow humans to refer to machines by name was introduced. This is is known as the *Domain Name System/Service or DNS*. In DNS, machines are grouped into a hierarchy of names, allowing related machines to be identified easily while giving enough flexibility for each machine to have several names and/or IP addresses associated with it.

At the top of the DNS hierarchy lie 13 "root" servers responsible for the notional "." highest level domain. These servers contain the details of the servers for the approved top-level domains (TLDs) such as "com", "gov", "mil", "uk", "tv" etc.

Each TLD has its own group of servers which contain pointers to the servers for the next layer down (e.g. ".ac.uk", ".co.uk", "microsoft.com") and so on until the servers at the bottom of the tree contain only details of the relationship between complete "Fully Qualified Domain Names" (FQDNs) for particular systems on the Internet, and their IP addresses.

Each network should have at least one DNS server to handle queries from its own machines, answer queries about its own domains or both.

When a machine needs to translate between a FQDN and the corresponding IP address, it queries its own DNS server (the local server) which either responds with the address (if it already knows it) or queries a more authoritative server for the domain. If the domain cannot be found, queries

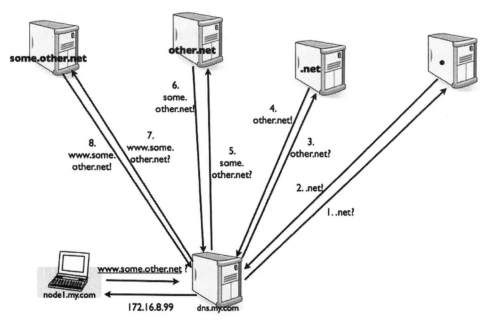

Figure 7.3   A DNS query in progress

will be sent to one of the root servers which will direct the local server to
the appropriate TLD server which directs the query down to a lower level,
and so on until the master server for the domain has been reached. Once
a server has received a response to a domain query, it stores a copy of the
response for a set period of time (determined by the domain master) for
future use. See Figure 7.3 for an example of this process.

In order to have the right to put entries into DNS, someone must claim
ownership of the domain. This usually involves buying, or more accurately
leasing, a domain name from a registrar recognised by DNS's governing
body – the Internet Corporation for Assigned Names and Numbers.[2] Once
the rights to use the name have been established, a record of "ownership"
of the domain name is placed into one of the international "WHOIS"
databases which list all domain names and their owners. Only then can DNS
entries be created in the appropriate DNS servers to allow the domain name
to be associated with the physical server(s) which host the services it offers.

---

[2]http://www.icann.org/.

For any enquiry, the WHOIS and DNS databases can provide significant information about the claimed ownership of any domain name and the associated IP addresses.

7.5 Internet applications

7.5.1 WWW

The World Wide Web was created at CERN in 1989 [5] by a British physicist, Tim Berners-Lee, attempting to solve the problem of keeping documents up to date within a large distributed organisation. His work drew on previous experiments with HyperText [35] systems and distributed information systems such as Gopher [3], but extended them to create a rich "information space" in which different media types and services could be accessed through a common user interface. The browser concept was quickly adopted and developed further by companies such as Netscape to produce a platform which was easy to use and thus appealed to a broad range of users with a wide range of knowledge and experience.

Strictly speaking, therefore, the world wide web is really a collection of services sitting on top of the wider Internet and accessible through a unified interface program. To most, though, the widespread use of the web has led to it becoming synonymous with the Internet as a whole, although there are many services available on the Internet which are not accessible through web browsers.

For the purposes of this discussion, we will focus on the two most popular components of the WWW: HTML and HTTP.

HTML is the HyperText Markup Language used to produce the web pages with which we have all become familiar. It is a way of describing the properties of elements on a page, allowing files to be embedded and links to other content to be defined using a simple scheme of "tags" which are written using a simple language designed to be as accessible as possible to non-programmers. A sample of HTML can be seen in Figure 7.4

All web pages consist of at least a page of HTML which may contain references to other resources such as hyperlinks or embedded objects. Hyperlinks are defined, within the HTML source, by `<a href=...>`

```
<html>
<head>
<title>A simple html example</title>
</head>
<body>
<p>This is some text in the HTML example and the
next bit will embed an image</p>
<img src=''images/myimage.jpg''/>
<p>Now this line contains a hy-
per<index>link</index>link to
<a href=''http://www.google.com''>google.com</a>
</p>
</body>
</html>
```

Figure 7.4   A sample of HTML used to compose a web page

tags, whereas embedded objects may be defined by tags such as `<img src=...>` for images and `<object>` for other objects such as embedded programs and movies.

Many of these tags contain references to data stored on the same server as the web page being interpreted, but some references will also be made to content held elsewhere. In these cases, the resource will be identified by a URL[3] which has the general form:

```
<scheme>://<user>:<password>@<server>:
   <port>/<resource-path>?<data>
```

where `<scheme>` is the protocol to be used to access the resource (e.g. http), `<user>` and `<password>` are the logon details to be sent with the request, `<server>` is the FQDN or IP address of the server to be contacted, `<port>` is the TCP port number on which the web server is listening (the default value is 80), `<resource-path>` is the full name of the resource as it will be understood by the server and `<data>` is any data to be sent to the server as part of the request. With the exception of `<scheme>`, `<server>` and `<resource-path>`, all of these elements are optional and may be omitted from the URL.

---

[3]Uniform Resource Locator.

At its simplest, then, a URL needs to be nothing more than

```
<scheme>://<server>/<resource>
    as in
```

```
http://www.google.co.uk/
```

In this example, the `<resource>` is the shortest one possible – a single /, denoting the default resource.

The default communications protocol for WWW transactions is the HyperText Transfer Protocol, HTTP. This is a very simple language defined in terms of basic operations required to allow information to be exchanged between two machines. By definition, it uses plain text for data presentation, but a variation known as HTTPS (for HTTP-Secure) provides encryption of data between client and server. Where the default port for HTTP is TCP port 80, HTTPS is usually found on TCP port 443 on the server.

Both versions have the same main functions which are defined by a few major commands:

- GET: the main HTTP command retrieves content from a specified resource.

- HEAD: retrieves information about a resource, without fetching any of the content. The HEAD data is also returned as part of the response to GET.

- POST: used to send data back to the server for processing.

- PUT: used to upload files/new content to the server.

Web browsers

When a web client (browser) connects to a server to retrieve a web page, it typically starts by issuing a GET command to retrieve the main HTML page. Once the HTML has been received, the browser will then issue a series of GETs and/or POSTs to retrieve embedded resources identified by the HTML. Thus a single web page, made up of multiple files, will require several requests from client to server.

Because Internet connections used to be very slow, early browsers were programmed to store copies of previously used resources locally in an area known as the *browser cache*. Not all material is cached, particularly if it has been accessed over a secure (HTTPS) connection, but even today most browsers still maintain a cache of previously accessed resources, which can prove invaluable to investigators looking for evidence of web activity. Files in the cache are no different from ordinary files, except that they have been created as a result of automatic download, which may fall into Chapter 5's "*AU*" category.

The exact location and name of this cache depends on the browser in use and the operating system. Users can also change the location of the cache by modifying browser options. Default cache folders tend to be well hidden, deep down in the user's filespace in areas that are notionally reserved for system and program use.

Most browsers also tend to keep a "history" of recently visited resources, so that popular or recently visited pages can be found from a "drop-down" list rather than forcing the user to remember a full URL. This history is usually stored in a file, somwhere near the cache, and includes date and time of last access. Again, this can be a useful source of information for an investigator.

The final piece of information which can routinely be recovered from web-browser storage is the collection of cookies built up over time. Cookies are small chunks of data stored by the browser, at the request of the web server. They are often used to prove that a user has logged into a web site, store details of items in a shopping basket, remember preferences set by the user, or even just to allow the web server to recognise returning users for statistical purposes. Without them, most of today's web applications would not work.

If the browser accepts and stores a cookie, it then presents the cookie data back to the server as part of subsequent requests. The server can then check the returned value against its own list of known cookies and perform appropriate processing.

Figure 7.5 shows the contents of a typical cookies. As with caches and history files, different browsers may use different storage mechanisms, but

Created	Domain	Expires	Name	Path	Value
231613802 99180999	scholar.google.co.uk	2038-01-17 19:14:07	GSP	/	ID=5406F79
229273537 89834601	eu.wiley.com	2010-04-07 15:05:37	utma	/	14086598...
229273537 89915299	eu.wiley.com	2008-10-07 03:05:37	utmz	/	14086598...

Figure 7.5   Contents of typical cookies from the author's web browser

will store cookies unless the user elects to override this behaviour. Within the cookie, we find the following fields:

- Created: the time and date of creation – encoded as the number of seconds since a reference date (usually midnight on Ist January, 1970).

- Domain: the domain to which the cookie should be returned. This may be a FQDN or an upper-level domain.

- Expires: the last valid date and time for the cookie. Some cookies may have infinite life, indicated by either a 0 or a large value here.

- Name: the name of the cookie as it is known to the server.

- Path: the starting point in the resource path for the server. When the browser accesses any resources at or below this path, the cookie will be sent to the server.

- Value: the data to be stored in the cookie. This may be numeric or alphabetic, and the meaning may not be obvious to anything except the receiving server.

Because cookies are stored in the browser's storage area, often in plain text or easily decodable files, they can be manipulated and deleted quite easily. In the author's experience, however, it is rare for someone to go to the trouble of manipulating cookies unless they wish to attempt to gain access to a restricted web resource which is protected by a user authentication system and uses cookies as proof that a correct login has occurred. In this situation, the criminal may copy a cookie from a legitimate user and then install it into his/her browser in order to impersonate that legitimate user.

7.5.2 E-mail

Electronic mail is still one of the most popular applications on the Internet and, for most people, can be split into two distinct operations: sending and collecting.

Sending e-mail

At the heart of Internet e-mail lies the SMTP (Simple Mail Transfer Protocol) [39], along with standard definitions of the format of mail messages [13]. These two standards laid the foundations for modern e-mail and, although there have been several refinements documented in later RFCs, they still enshrine the main principles of operation of e-mail sending on the Internet today.

SMTP defines a mechanism which allows mail software to either deliver messages directly to the receiving system, especially if it is local, or to pass undeliverable messages on to "smart" hosts which act as intermediate relays. These smart hosts may also pass mail along to another relay, creating a chain of mail hosts, until the message eventually arrives at a mail server that can deliver the message to the target system. In DNS, most domains have relays defined through the use of Mail eXchange (MX) records, and these machines are usually the only ones which can be reached via port 25, the SMTP port.

As the mail passes through each relay, the relay adds an extra line of information to the top of the message, giving details of where it was received from, the time of receipt and where it seems to be going. In this way, each e-mail transmitted over SMTP picks up a set of "headers" which contain complete details of its journey across the Internet (see Figure 7.6).

By default, SMTP relays will hold e-mail and attempt to deliver it for a period of up to seven days before deciding that the receiving network is unreachable and returning it to the point of origin with an error message. Of course, if the receiving network does not exist (i.e. has no valid DNS entry or IP address), the server will reject it immediately.

Amongst the weaknesses in the definitions of SMTP and mail message format is the requirement for mail clients (sending software) to generate

```
Delivered-To: xxxxxxxxxxxx@gmail.com
Received: by 10.142.224.1 with SMTP id w1cs78057wfg;
     Wed, 5 Mar 2008 16:56:32 -0800 (PST)
Received: by 10.82.182.1 with SMTP id e1mr6469630buf.21.1204764990299;
     Wed, 05 Mar 2008 16:56:30 -0800 (PST)
Return-Path: <FreemanlocomotionHurley@dispatch.com>
Received: from xxxxxxx.xxxxxxxxx.co.uk (xxxxxxx.xxxxxxxxx.co.uk [212.67.202.165])
     by mx.google.com with ESMTP id h6si1305423nfh.30.2008.03.05.16.56.29;
     Wed, 05 Mar 2008 16:56:30 -0800 (PST)
Received-SPF: neutral (google.com: 212.67.202.165 is neither permitted nor
          denied by best guess record for domain of
          xxxxxx@xxxx.com) client-ip=212.67.202.165;
Authentication-Results: mx.google.com; spf=neutral (google.com: 212.67.202.165 is
                neither permitted nor denied by best guess record for
                domain of xxxxxx@xxxx.com)
                smtp.mail=xxxxxx@xxxx.com
Received: from [76.76.168.165] (helo=hp22952133567)
by xxxxxxx.xxxxxxxxx.co.uk with smtp (Exim 4.54)
id 1JX4PM-0006QG-St
for xxxxxxx@xxxxxx.net; Thu, 06 Mar 2008 00:56:29 +0000
Message-ID: 149b501c87f462b28c6b00a01a8c0@HP22952133567
From: "Myles Cervantes" <xxxxxx@xxxx.com>
To: <xxxxxxx@xxxxxx.net>
Subject: your exclusive watches rolex
Date: Wed, 5 Mar 2008 20:47:56 +0800
MIME-Version: 1.0
Content-Type: text/plain;
format=flowed;
charset="iso-8859-1";
reply-type=original
Content-Transfer-Encoding: 7bit
X-Priority: 3
X-MSMail-Priority: Normal
X-Mailer: Microsoft Outlook Express 6.00.2800.1106
X-MimeOLE: Produced By Microsoft MimeOLE V6.00.2800.1106

Discover Our Range of Luxury Rolex Timepieces for Men and Women...
ALL at low prices!

http://scamsite.com/
```

Figure 7.6   A sample e-mail showing full headers

the "From:", "To:" and several other headers themselves. As a result, much of the information in these critical headers can be forged – a property which is exploited to good effect by many of those who send unsolicited commercial e-mail (UCE or Spam).

For this reason, it is considered essential to be able to inspect the full headers (i.e. those inserted by the relay hosts) in order to determine the true origins of any e-mail. Unfortunately, most modern e-mail clients hide these headers from end users as they are considered confusing and irrelevant. However, it is usually possible to get the mail software to disclose the headers with a little bit of persuasion. If this cannot be done in the software directly, the headers are almost always present in the file in which received e-mail is stored.

Collecting e-mail

The advent of personal computers in the 1980s, leading to the fulfilment of Pournelle's law, led to a situation where delivery to a local server was no longer sufficient to allow users to work with e-mail efficiently. Either all desktop machines had to be capable of receiving SMTP, which could lead to problems if machines were switched off for prolonged periods, or a mechanism which allowed users to collect their e-mail on demand needed to be devised.

In 1984, the first such system was published as RFC918 [41], defining the "Post Office Protocol" as a means for client software to collect e-mail from mailboxes held on a central server. This has evolved into POP-3 [34], which extends the original functionality to support more advanced features.

A further development lies in the design and implementation of IMAP [12] (Internet Message Access Protocol) which, in addition to allowing retrieval and deletion of e-mail on the server, allows users to create and manipulate folders for e-mail storage on the server as well.

From an investigative point of view, the retrieval mechanism has little or no effect on the content of the messages retrieved, but may be significant if we need to examine a mailbox which is still active on a server. If we know which retrieval protocol was in use, we can ensure that checks are carried out for all features supported by that protocol.

Other standards

In addition to these open standards, vendors such as AOL[4] and Microsoft have their own communication standards for mail sending and retrieval. The proprietary, closed, nature of these standards means that little detail

---

[4]America OnLine.

about them is available, but messages sent and received through these systems usually have to cross the public Internet at some point in their lives, meaning that they may still carry SMTP headers.

7.5.3 Chatrooms and chat fora

Many web site and Internet communities/social network sites offer areas where users can chat to each other in real-time, or near real-time. Since these chatroom or forum systems are web based they leave similar traces to web pages and, on the server, there is usually a record of the IP address used to post messages along with time and login information associated with each message. Users can adopt any identity they wish, but ultimately the messages they exchange can be traced back to the originating machines through IP addresses.

7.5.4 Instant messengers and peer-to-peer (P2P) software

Instant messengers, such as AOL messenger, GoogleTalk, MSN messenger, ICQ, IRC and Jabber operate in a manner similar to peer-to-peer (P2P) file sharing software such as eMule, Gnutella, BitTorrent and others. Although generally falling under the heading of P2P, they actually tend to operate in either a client-server mode or a true peer-to-peer mode.

In client-server mode a single "exchange" node receives messages from one user and forwards them to the others in the conversation. In this situation, the client machine may have some logs of who was contacted and, if the examiner is lucky, even a log file containing details of the data exchanged. It is unlikely, however, to contain any IP information other than the address of the server which was acting as the gateway for the conversation.

In true peer-to-peer mode, one or more machines may act as a "telephone directory" (also known as a "Super Node"), listing those users who are currently online and, where file sharing is involved, the resources they are offering out to the rest of the community. Once the client has consulted the directory, direct contact is established with the other party in the conversation (much more like a real telephone call), and both ends of the conversation need to know the other's IP address in order to exchange data.

In both situations, there is no requirement for the software to record anything at all about the data exhange, but many programs do keep records of recent activity, including IP addresses in use at the time. Again, if an IP address and/or a username can be found, then it may be possible to carry out tracing through liaison with Internet Service Providers and server owners.

In some systems, the Super Nodes are not fixed points, but are elected periodically by the other peer-to-peer clients on the network, thus they can be difficult to identify and will change over time.

7.5.5 Anonymising techniques

Proxies   In many networks, traffic is routinely diverted via a "proxy server" which sits between the local network and the wider Internet. These proxies can help network management by providing two services: filtering out unwanted content (i.e. acting as censors to prevent access to unwanted or illegal material) and acting as large local caches of material that is regularly accessed by a large number of users. By keeping copies of material on the local network, the amount of traffic generated on the Internet can be reduced and local users can be given faster access to the most used material.

From the point of view of a server, a proxy looks like just another client and, apart from some which disclose their nature in request headers, cannot be distinguished from any other client program. As a result, a network of 200 machines operating through a proxy will appear as a single IP address to anything outside the local network.

For network investigators, this poses several challenges, not least because of the existence of *Anonymising Proxies*, which are designed to hide all details of the point of origin of requests sent through the proxy. Requests made via such a proxy can be traced back to the proxy, but rarely, if ever, back to the real origin.

Onion skin routing   Proxies act as simple relays, using the protocols already in existence on the Internet for communications, and it is (in theory at least) possible to intercept and monitor communications which use these protocols. There is another way of creating anonymous communications channels which use encryption to carry any data at all from one point to another, without the intermediaries being able to read the content of any messages.

This method uses a chain of relays, each of which has its own encryption/decryption in place. The sender determines which nodes are going to act as relays for it and builds a pre-determined route. It then encrypts the data to be sent using the keys for the relays, in the right order, to create a series of wrappers or "skins" around the data, and sends the message to the first relay. This relay removes its "skin" to find the next layer of encryption and the address of the next relay to send to.

Each node is, therefore, only aware of the node that sent the message to it, and the node it is sending to. Relay nodes cannot read the message because it has been encrypted with another node's key. Only the target node has the right key to decrypt the final message.

The description of this as "Onion Skin Routing" comes from an analogy with peeling an onion, layer by layer, until the core is exposed. The transmitted data are the core, the skins are the encryption and routing addresses. "Pass the parcel" would be an equally good name.

Interception of a message at a node yields nothing more than the previous and next nodes and the encrypted data to be sent to the next node. Identification of origin and target at intermediate nodes is, therefore, impossible without extremely powerful decryption systems (see section 6.1.5 for a discussion of encryption).

7.5.6 Web "drops"

A final twist comes from the use of web-based e-mail systems. Normally, any messages sent through these systems are subject to the same rules as any other mail sent using SMTP, although it may be difficult to determine which machine was used to access the web mail server.

In recent times, it has been seen that some criminals/terrorists have started to use webmail in a novel way, exploiting one of the features to exchange messages without sending them. This makes it difficult to show that a message has been sent or received.

Instead of typing in a message and sending it, as would be the normal case, these users are creating messages and saving them in the online system as "drafts" which are stored to be sent at some later date and time. Their accomplices can log on to the same e-mail account, using WWW access, from anywhere in the world, to read and edit messages in the same way. Thus, instant communication between two conspirators on opposite sides of the world can be achieved, without any data being explicitly transmitted from one to the other.

In principle, this is similar to the old spy trick of leaving secret messages in hollow tree stumps or other "dead letter drops" for collection by another agent at some time in the future.

8
Mobile Devices

One of the effects of Moore's law [32] has been a massive reduction in component size alongside reductions in power requirement and price. This has created opportunities for the development of low-cost portable personal technology which has proved to be very attractive to the mass market. Devices such as mobile phones, digital cameras, digital media players, satellite navigation systems and personal digital assistants have all seen significant take-up since their introduction, and it is probably fair to say that a majority of homes has at least one of these devices.

At heart, each of these devices is, in essence, a micro-computer and follows the same principles of operation as discussed elsewhere in this book, but the operating systems and applications on these devices are often highly specialised, and may operate in such a way that data extraction and interpretation is less simple than with general-purpose computers.

8.1 Mobile phones and PDAs

Personal Digital Assistants started life as replacements for FiloFax-style paper-based personal organisers in the 1990s, but their functionality has largely been supplanted by equivalent functions which are now offered in even "low-end" mobile phones. As a result, although there are still many PDAs in existence, this section will concentrate on evidential opportunities presented by mobile phones. Generally speaking, with the exception of

Digital Forensics: Digital Evidence in Criminal Investigation   Angus M. Marshall
© 2008 John Wiley & Sons, Ltd

communications data, the material available from PDAs will be similar to that found on phones, and many phones and PDAs are built around the same mobile operating system (e.g. Windows CE/PocketPC/Mobile, Palm OS, Linux & Symbian).

Because these devices are designed to be portable and in-use for prolonged periods, they are battery powered. Older devices used standard replaceable power cells, but modern units are equipped with internal rechargeable batteries which can power the device for several days at a time between recharges.

The sheer number of different physical connections used on these devices over the years, and the different power standards adopted by different manufacturers mean that it is vital for anyone seizing equipment of this type to at least attempt to find the power adapter and interface cables associated with it. This is not always possible, so any good examination facility should have kits similar to that shown in Figure 8.1 to allow connections to the majority of devices. Fortunately, the emergence of the USB standard means that more and more manufacturers are electing to use standard cables instead of their older proprietary connectors.

We can consider these devices to have three main storage areas (two for PDAs) which may be present: internal memory, internal memory and SIM card memory (not on PDAs).

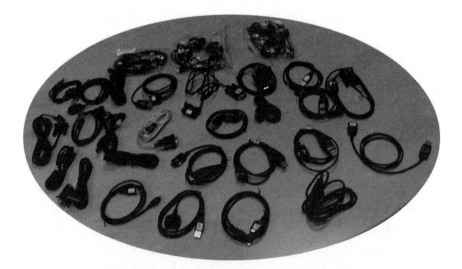

Figure 8.1 A typical set of interface cables found in a mobile device examination kit

Removable memory

Most modern devices have a slot where a memory storage card can be inserted into the device to expand the storage space available and allow data to be exchanged with other devices. These memory cards conform to the same standards as for other devices with removable storage, and usually use the same standard FAT[1] filesystem found in those devices. As a result, the examination of the memory cards can be carried out using standard forensic data examination tools, and the principles and mechanisms described in preceding chapters apply. Care must be taken, however, to ensure that the examiner is aware of how the device's operating system handles the MAC timestamps and file deletion, as portable devices may exhibit unusual behaviours (e.g. not setting access times, or completely erasing data when a file is deleted), leading to different interpretations of their contents and activity.

Fortunately, because these storage devices are designed to be moved between hosts, they do not lose data when power is removed and can be treated as hard discs for examination purposes, although an adapter such as that shown in Figure 8.2 may be required to allow the software to read the contents.

Internal memory

The internal memory of a portable device needs to fulfil two functions: it must operate as both the device's primary memory for program execution, and as a filesystem for data storage. Depending on how the device has been programmed, there may be distinct areas within memory set aside for this, or it may move memory from one use to another on demand.

Exactly how this memory is organised may not be visible to an external user and the distinction between RAM and ROM may not be obvious. Memory organisation may be particularly difficult to determine if the device provides an emulation mode, where it appears to be a removable

---

[1] File Allocation Table.

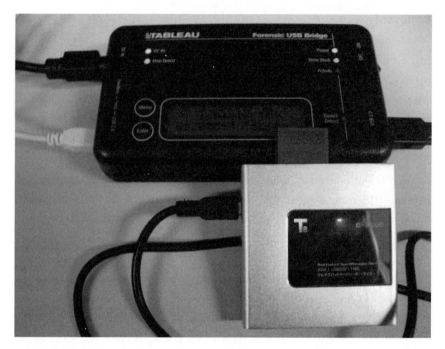

Figure 8.2 A multi-format removable memory card reader connected via a forensic bridge write-blocker

storage device when connected to a general purpose computer, as it may attempt to provide a single unified view of all storage areas as if they were a single device.

Many devices provide two different modes of operation when connected to a computer: one for synchronisation of personal data (e.g. diaries, e-mail, notes etc.) and one for transfer of data files. It is likely that neither of these modes actually provides a true picture of the contents of internal memory and it may be necessary to either dismantle the device and connect it to specialist diagnostic equipment, or to install a data recovery program on the device.

Installation of the data recovery program, of course, violates ACPO Principle 1 [2] (Chapter 4), because it entails modifying the state of the device. However, ACPO Principle 2 allows for this to happen when the person performing the installation and examination is qualified to provide an explanation of their actions and how they may have affected any recovered evidence.

It should be noted that the internal memory of these devices generally needs to be faster and more flexible than removable storage and tends to use the same type of technology as that found in desktop and laptop computers. When power is lost, the contents of the memory will also be lost, although recent studies have suggested [19] that it may be possible to access data in volatile memory after a period of a few minutes, or even longer if the memory is chilled. This result has not, at the time of writing, been fully validated as an acceptable method for handling volatile storage so should be considered an avenue of last resort.

SIM cards and mobile telephony

[Note: the discussion in this section relates mainly to the GSM (Global System for Mobile Communications) network with some relevance to the UMTS (Universal Mobile Telecommunications System) network. These are the standards across Europe. Other network standards are used in other parts of the world.]

Finally, in the case of mobile phones, we can consider the SIM (Subscriber Identity Module) or U-SIM (UMTS Subscriber Identity Module) card (Figure 8.3). These cards are part of a general family of "smart" cards [40] or UICCs (Universal Integrated Circuit Cards) which contain small quantities of memory and/or processing capability.

For simplicity, we will concentrate on the SIM card, but USIM provides similar features, albeit in a more advanced way.

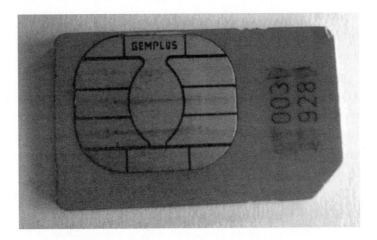

Figure 8.3   A standard small-format modern SIM card

As the name suggests, a SIM card provides a way of associating a handset with a subscriber to allow access to the mobile phone network. In order for the network to know where to route call data to, it requires both a logical and physical address (equivalent to the IP and MAC addresses used in the IP suite (see Section 7.3). In the mobile phone network, the physical address is the IMSI (International Mobile Subscriber Identity) which is unique to the SIM and programmed in during manufacture. The logical address is the telephone number associated with the SIM through a database which maps the telephone number to the IMSI.

Thus, in order to connect a call, the network matches the telephone number dialled to the IMSI and the call can be routed through to the IMSI's current location.

Another physical identifier exists within the handset, in the form of the IMEI (International Mobile Equipment Identity), and this can be used to identify the handset in use with a particular IMSI or to inform the network that the handset is not permitted to connect if it has been reported stolen.

The SIM standard provides for several small storage areas within the module. Some of the more useful of these, from an investigative perspective, tend to be the following:

- Operator data: an area reserved for the network provider to identify which network services and restrictions are in force for the subscriber. For example, this area may list networks which must NOT be connected to, which networks to look for when abroad, whether or not the user is permitted to use the handset abroad etc. One entry which may be of interest in this category is that of the cell in which the handset was last switched off.

- Personal data: an area for storage of data created by the SIM user. Typically this may hold their personal address/phone book, short-code dialling numbers, calls made and received and SMS (text) messages sent and received.

- PIN/PUK status: this records whether or not a PIN (Personal Identification Number) is required to activate the SIM along with how many times an incorrect PIN has been presented. When the number of incorrect

PIN entries exceeds a threshold, the user must enter the Personal Unlock Key (PUK) set by the network operator. Again, there is a fixed number of attempts available for entry of the PUK. If this is exceeded, the SIM becomes effectively unusable. Examiners should take care to check PIN/PUK status before attempting any other access to the card.

A sample SIM card report can be found in Appendix C.

Cell-site analysis

Another fruitful area of investigation involving mobile phones is that of cell-site analysis. This attempts to plot the location where a phone is, or has been used, based on properties of the mobile phone network itself. The GSM network is made up of a network of transmitter/receiver masts, each of which provides coverage for at least one cell. A single mast may operate in all directions at once, or may have directional antennae providing signals in different directions. In rural and/or areas of low population density the masts are usually a few km apart, whereas in urban/highly populated areas the masts need to be much closer together (a few hundred m at most) in order to be able to cope with the number of handsets in the area.

As a handset moves from location to location, it polls the network to determine which mast can provide the best service to it. As a "better" cell is detected, the network switches the handset from the current cell to the new one (the process of "cell handover"), ensuring that calls in progress are not interrupted. Thus, the handset is always aware of which cell it is located in, and the network always knows, approximately, where the handset is based on the antenna in use and the signal strength (which gives a guide to distance from the mast). Cells are typically drawn as idealised hexagons, but in reality the shape of each cell is affected by attenuation of signal strength caused by environmental influences such as trees, hills and buildings.

By mapping signal strengths around a mast, it is possible to predict where cell handover will occur for each network and, if a log of cells used by a handset can be obtained, produce an approximate map of the route taken by the handset.

When a handset is switched off, it signals this fact to the network and both the handset and network record the cell in which it was last active.

When calls are made, the network produces a *Call Detail Record* (CDR) for billing purposes. Usually this contains, at least, the starting and ending cells for the call along with called number and duration. Although not necessarily a complete list of all cells used during the call, it may be possible to estimate the movement of the handset by plotting signal strengths and predicting cell handovers.

The handset's constant interaction with the network is, possibly, the biggest threat to continuity of evidence, as any interaction post-discovery may result in alteration of the device's contents.

The ACPO Good Practice Guide for Computer Based Electronic Evidence [2] contains detailed advice on the handling of mobile phones. Use of Faraday cages/bags is strongly recommended for the seizure, transport and examination of these devices, but it should be remembered that if a phone cannot contact a cell, it will continue to broadcast using stronger and stronger signals until it either finds a cell or its power supply is exhausted. Since the networks use different frequencies (GSM uses 900 MHz, 1800 MHz, 950 MHz, 1900 MHz, 400 MHz and 450 MHz depending on country), it should not be assumed that all Faraday cages/bags will isolate the handset from all networks. Different Faraday cages/bags will have different levels of permeability for the various frequencies.

8.2 GPS

GPS, the Global Positioning System, uses a network of satellites in orbit around the planet. Each satellite has a unique identity and a well-defined orbital path combined with an accurate clock. Each satellite broadcasts information about the current time and its orbit.

By identifying the satellites "visible" from any point on the planet and performing a calculation based on the data sent by the satellites, a GPS receiver can calculate exactly where it is above the surface of the planet.

Although designed originally for military use, GPS technology has reached the consumer market, where a typical receiver costs around the

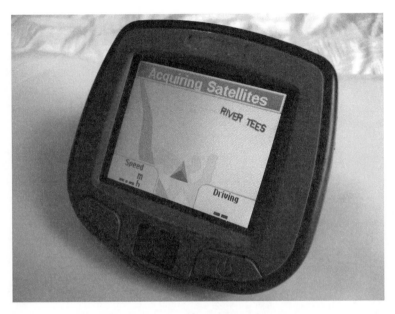

Figure 8.4   A typical consumer GPS unit for use in-car

same as a PDA. The use of this technology has become very popular with drivers, walkers, sailors and amateur pilots as an aid to navigation, so it is becoming increasingly common for computer crime units to be asked to examine these devices for possible evidence.

GPS devices (Figure 8.4) are showing signs of convergence with PDA technology, with some GPS units now having media player facilities, the ability to connect to mobile phones via Bluetooth, WiFi potential, and general-purpose storage functions as well.

Examination of GPS equipment can be more problematic than examination of phones. Some systems use versions of the operating systems designed for PDAs, while others are based on entirely proprietary navigation software.

If interrogation of the device can be carried out, though, it may be possible to retrieve navigation data about the point of last use, lists of favourite places and pre-planned routes, in addition to other usage information which depends on the other features available on the device.

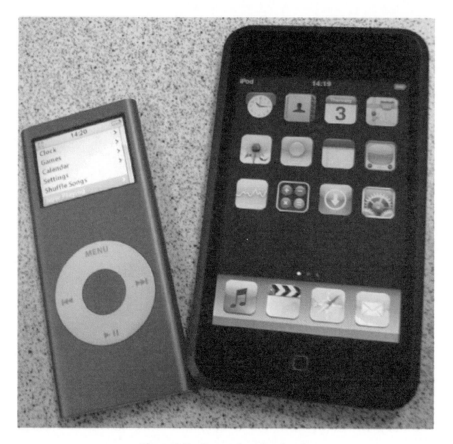

Figure 8.5   Personal media players

8.3 Other personal technology

Most people now own at least a few other examples of personal technology
in the form of digital cameras, media players (Figure 8.5) etc. On the
whole, these devices are single-function but can operate as external storage
devices when connected to more powerful computers. Some, however, are
appearing with the convergent properties described above. In addition to
their main functions, they offer PDA-type functionality, WiFi connectivity
etc. with all the evidential opportunites and investigative problems that
those features create.

9

Intelligence

9.1 Device usage

Because digital devices are used in all walks of life from education, through business to entertainment and other personal uses, they have become a rich source of intelligence information.

In this context, intelligence relates to information which may assist us by giving some clues about the background, intent, state of mind, actions or network of contacts related to the person whose device is being examined.

Depending on the nature of the device there will be greater or lesser amounts of information available, with differing levels of ease of recovery.

For example, a desktop PC is likely to be a rich information source containing much in the way of historical data. Because its storage system is well defined and understood, and constrained by the need to allow components to be interchangeable between different systems, it is relatively easy to recover data from the system. A mobile phone, however, as a device which has a lower requirement to allow exchange of hardware components, although still a potentially rich source of data, poses a bigger challenge for data recovery.

Assuming data can be recovered, though, we can use the techniques described earlier in this book to analyse those data and build up a picture of the user(s) of the device in question.

Digital Forensics: Digital Evidence in Criminal Investigation   Angus M. Marshall
© 2008 John Wiley & Sons, Ltd

9.1.1 Timeline analysis

By examining the timestamp meta-data it is possible to construct a timeline of activity on the machine, possibly going back over a period of several weeks or months, to establish the normal pattern of usage, if one exists. A timeline of this type can help to identify events which fall outside the usual pattern, and may be indicative of some abnormal external influence on the user. Alternatively, timeline analysis can be used to predict when certain events may re-occur.

The greater the number of files on the system, in total, the more likely a timeline is to be accurate and useful. Devices that are used only infrequently tend to have too little data for a regular pattern to be detectable.

9.1.2 Stored data

Data stored on a system, of course, represent the outcome of some activity on that system.

By examining the locations and content of data files, it is possible to determine the nature of the activities performed. Data held in the web browser cache may give an indication of personal interests, business activities, hobbies, research, planning etc. and help to build up a picture of the type of person who uses the system. If this information is combined with the timeline information, it is possible to distinguish between work and leisure activities to some extent.

Information held in stored files may give an indication, not only of who we are dealing with, but about past activites and plans for the future.

9.1.3 Data exchange

Data exchange really relates to interactions with other people or systems. Received e-mails, participation in social networking sites (Facebook, MySpace, Bebo and others), SMS messages, phone calls, faxes, etc. all have the potential to allow us to identify the personal network of the

individual under investigation. This may lead us to co-conspirators, potential or past victims, or those who have been planning to make the system's
user a target.

9.2 Profiling and cyberprofiling

In order to build up a clear picture of the user of the system, and their
contacts, we need to turn to the world of profiling, both criminal and
geographic.

Over the years, various criminological theories have been developed,
which assist in predicting properties of criminals and related crimes based
on observed patterns of activity. In this section, some results from the
2005/06 EPSRC-funded Cyberprofiling project [51] are presented for consideration.

This project examined how the principles and methods of "mainstream"
profiling could be applied to observed Internet activity, with a particular
emphasis on the detection and prediction of patterns of criminal activity
in order to prevent such activity.

Background

Consideration of Routine Activity Theory [10], and Marauders and Commuters [7] suggests that, for a crime to happen, a motivated criminal and
a suitable victim must be in an appropriate environment, in the absence
of a suitable guardian, at the same time. Furthermore, the criminal and/or
victim may have to travel to the location in order for the crime to be
committed.

Consideration of these two models leads to the composite theory developed in the cyberprofiling work.

It is not always necessary for the criminal and victim to be in the same
location at the same time. Instead, the criminal must have passed through
the location at some time up to, and including, the point when the victim
moves into the location, and must have deposited some means of launching
an attack agains the victim at that location during this time (Figure 9.1).

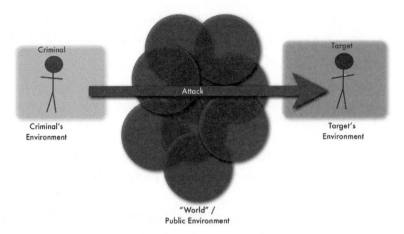

Figure 9.1   "Real world" crime

This modified model allows us to include consideration of remotely triggered attacks such as bombs, which may be deposited hours or days in advance.

In accepting this model, in order to allow it to be applied to online activity, we need to consider the elements of "cyberspace" which provide analogues to the "real world" concepts embodied above.

9.2.1 Factors in online crime

Motivation

The concept of motivation is, perhaps, the most difficult one to analyse.

For our purposes, a motivator may be external or internal to the criminal. For this analysis, it is considered to be a property of the criminal, which can be either active or passive, deliberate or accidental. Indeed, the motivation process may, itself, be a criminal or unwanted act which our model aims to represent.

Other factors

The other factors are similar to those found in other, "conventional" crimes. In his "cyberpunk" novels, William Gibson [16] created a useful way to refer to the world of computer networks, and human activity within them, as "cyberspace". Derived from this is the concept of "meatspace", as a shorthand for "the real, physical world" where flesh and blood exist.

In cyberspace crime, the criminal is still a meatspace person, and the ultimate victim is likely to be a meatspace person, even if the attack is to a machine, as machines only exist to provide services to people (see Chapter 2).

The environments being considered will have both cyberspace and meatspace elements. For example, a computer can be secured physically, under lock and key, and also by the use of security software devices within the realm of cyberspace. Similarly we can argue that guardians can be persons performing the guardianship function, or software and hardware elements having a similar role. For example, we can consider a user-authentication system, a network firewall and a software virus filter as forms of cyber-guardian.

In meatspace a witness is normally considered as a person, but modern forensic science embraces, perhaps slightly reluctantly, the concept of a "Silent Witness": an object that was present at the time, and can be examined to provide some form of testimony about events or persons present. In cyberspace there can be many forms of silent witness that gather computerised evidence and traces of the activity in that world.

9.2.2 Analysis

In meatspace, once data about a crime have been gathered, from a variety of sources, a thorough and comprehensive analysis may then take place. This analysis performs a vital role in developing an understanding of the circumstances of the attack, and demonstrates any relationship which exists between that and previous attacks, perhaps giving an outline as to possible future developments in terms of attack evolution.

These data also perform a key role in allowing for the development of profiles, of the victim, of the perpetrator, and of the illicit activity.

The profiler, applying victimology principles [52], is able to provide an opinion of any particularly "attractive" properties which the victim possesses, which may predispose them to becoming the victim of an attack.

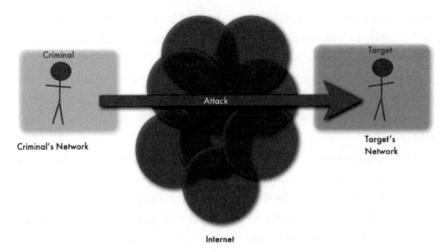

Figure 9.2   Internet model of crime

To the same ends, similar opinions can be produced about the criminal entity and the activity.

In cyberspace, the criminal needs to posses sufficient levels of motivation to attack the target, and the necessary knowledge/experience/background to be able to do so. The nature of the crime may demonstrate the likely "career" path of the perpetrator.

Environmental factors are important aspects in the determination of whether a crime will succeed, or the elements supporting crime, but the nature of the Internet, as a network of networks, allows us to subdivide the environment more easily than can be done with meatspace. Without exception, we can consider the totality of cyberspace to be made up of three elements: the criminal's network, the victim's network and the Internet connecting them. The Internet thus represents a transport mechanism to allow the criminal to gain access to the victim's network (Figure 9.2). This is, as far as can be determined, consistent with both Routine Activity Theory and the Marauders and Commuters model.

9.3 Evaluating online crime: automating the model

One of the goals of the Cyberprofiling project [48] was to automate elements of the profiling and modelling process described above.

Examination of the model suggests that we can express the various elements affecting the results of the crime as parameters to an equation which can indicate the likelihood of the success of an attack through the different environments.

The first factor is the Criminal Expertise Ce which reflects how skillful and/or experienced the criminal is. Similarly we can express a factor for how much expertise the victim has. The network environments themselves are largely irrelevant, except for the constraints placed upon users in those environments. Thus we consider the guardianship in the environments, expressed as the two factors Cg and Vg. We also need a factor to encapsulate the nature of the attack, which will encompass its novelty and other elements that contribute to success; this can be denoted by A. Finally, the freedom with which the criminal can deliver the attack from his "home" network to the victim's network, across the Internet, can be included as a factor, C_f, that represents the Criminal's freedom to operate over the network (this may be considered to be the inverse of the guardianship of the Internet; in most cases the guardianship will be negligible as the Internet was not designed to be an inherently secure system).

We can combine these factors to generate a figure for the attack likelihood L.

$$L = \frac{Ce \times C_f \times A}{Ve \times (Cg)^x \times Vg}$$

Also included is the additional modifier, x, which can reflect the importance of guardianship on the miscreants. This modifier is an arbitrary value, which is used to denote the importance in the formula of the guardianship of the criminal.

Values within this formula are identified as being on a sliding scale from 1 to 5, with 1 being a lower level and 5 a higher level. The resultant values within the formula denote the likelihood of success of a particular venture. Using an arbitrary value for x of 2 will give a denominator of up to 625. This is felt to be as high as is required; however, where a value of this size is present, it indicates that defences are strong, and only a determined criminal with a high degree of skill would be likely to succeed.

The range of L is thus 1/625 (highly unlikely to succeed) to 125/1 (almost guaranteed success).

9.4 Application of the formula to case studies

In order to fully understand the model and method of assessment, it is worthwhile taking some time to outline a number of possible scenarios, both Internet and closed system based.

9.4.1 iPod fraud

Sale of an iPod on auction sites such as eBay is commonplace. As such, it is a worthwhile area of focus. The vendor appears to list an iPod for sale for 99 ¢, and a potential purchaser develops an interest in the item for sale. On closer inspection, usually after the sale has been concluded, the purchaser is found to have merely bought information. In this case it is typically an e-book similar to "How to buy an iPod".

From this, we can deduce several things. Firstly, on delivery, the victim receives apparently "misdescribed" goods. The criminal has, in fact, utilised an excessive description to mask the inaccuracy of the actual sale, without actually breaking any of the written rules of the online environment. This form of attack is very commonplace and, according to our observations of complaints about it, widely considered to be a moral crime, if not a crime as defined by statute or rule-book.

From observations, it seems that the victims are typically younger members of the community, at least in terms of experience of participating in the community, and frequently below the age permitted by user agreements.

Applying the earlier formula to this scenario, it is possible to attribute values to the "scam". We can assign the value of 3 to the expertise of the criminal (Ce), a moderate level. The value is deduced not only from the technical ability of the miscreant, but also the organisational ability and understanding of the manner of operation of the auction site.

Such cases often start with the criminal operating from a bedroom, within a home network, therefore with a low level of security, with a typical value of Cg of 1.

As many of the users of the sites are young and relatively naíve, the Ve value is low at 1.

Again, the victim of the attack is on a home network, the guardianship levels Vg are low, with a value of 1. The attack type, A, is classed as 3, a moderate level. Attacks of this type require a certain understanding of the rules of the community, and ways in which they can be subverted. It should be noted that the level of the attack, in this case, is not dependent on the level of the criminal.

Cf represents the security of the Internet as inherently insecure, therefore the high value of 5 appropriately shows that the criminal has virtually unlimited freedom to deliver the attack to the victim.

We can apply these values to determine an indicator of success likelihood:

$$L = \frac{3 \times 5 \times 3}{1 \times (1)^2 \times 1}$$
$$L = 45$$

A rating of 45 represents a significant likelihood of success, being far closer to the maximum value of 125, which represents almost guaranteed success. This is borne out by the observation that this attack re-occurs frequently on the web sites which we have observed.

9.4.2 (Distributed) denial of service attack

Consider, next, a Denial of Service (DoS) Attack. In this situation, a criminal uses Internet-connected devices to flood one or more servers with requests. The result of this flood is that the server(s) in question are overwhelmed and no longer able to service legitimate requests from real users. Such attacks are commonly associated with blackmail attempts (for example in the case of online gambling sites) or activists protesting about some issue (e.g. attacks on the McDonald's web sites during G7/G8 protests).

In order to launch such an attack, the criminal needs to be quite familiar with the ways in which such attacks work. Thus we would rate him/her as $Ce = 5$. The network launching the attack has no mechanisms in place to prevent such an attack escaping and is rated as $Cg = 1$. The Internet, as usual, allows the attack to be delivered with minimal controls. $Cf = 4$, representing the fact that there are some restrictions in place, but very few.

The victim has little opportunity to prevent the attacks, and probably has little experience of them, giving $Ve = 2$, and finally, the victim's network must be moderately open to this attack, in spite of firewalls and anti-virus precautions, as it uses the same mechanisms as legitimate network traffic. $Vg = 3$, therefore.

Applying the formula gives the following:

$$L = \frac{5 \times 4 \times 2}{2 \times (1)^2 \times 3}$$
$$L = 6.66$$

The figure of $L = 6.66$, aside from being pleasingly biblical in nature, estimates that the DoS attack has only a moderate likelihood of success. This, again, reflects the reality that most networks now have some protection against this type of attack entering them.

9.4.3 CD piracy

As a final example, we turn to a "closed system" crime. In this case, that of a "low-level" copyright violator. Typically, these criminals use cheap home PCs equipped with multiple CD/DVD writers to produce copies of music, movies and software for sale at public markets or on internet sites.

The equipment is easy to use and the raw materials are freely available on the high street. The criminal, therefore, needs little experience or skill and can be rated as $Ce = 1$. The criminal does, however, need somewhere to conduct the copying activity and runs the risk of observation. Since the majority of this activity happens at home, we have rated it as having moderate guardianship with $Cg = 3$. The victim, in this case, is the industry that produces legitimate copies of the material. This includes multi-national companies with dedicated teams of investigators, working with law enforcement agencies. As a result, we consider the victim's expertise rating to be quite high; $Ve = 4$. For the same reasons, the victim's guardianship is quite high; $Vg = 4$. For the crime to succeed, the criminal must make sales, and this requires activity in a public place which may be subject to observation; Cf, the freedom to move, is thus reduced and we rate it as

$C_f = 3$. Finally, the attack type is low. It requires minimum special equipment and is understood to be commonplace; $A = 2$.

$$L = \frac{1 \times 3 \times 2}{4 \times (3)^2 \times 3}$$
$$L = 1/18 = 0.056$$

Once more, this evaluation of the crime as unlikely to succeed is borne out by experiences of the successful investigation and prosecution of "lower-level" copyright violators of the type described.

9.5 From success estimates to profiling

The method proposed above provides a forward-calculation method based on values for each of the elements constituting the incident or attack. In reality, we are likely to be faced with unknowns. However, it is possible to provide an estimate for the value of L and, using values for the elements which can be identified, the calculation can be reversed to provide estimated, values for the unknowns.

This leads us towards the production of profiles for the unknown elements. Each of the values C_f, Ce, Cg, Ve, Vg, A is a composite, representing the totality of each of the elements in the incident. It is proposed that it is possible to produce these figures using appropriate calculations based on scalar measures of properties of each of these elements.

For example, the value A is likely to be composed from measures of attack novelty, attack prevalence, attack severity etc.

The primary challenge remains, though, to determine what the parameters of each element are, and how they should be combined to allow both forward and backward profiling to be performed. A secondary challenge exists in the consideration of whether or not this proposed automatic profiling system can be applied back to the "real world".

9.6 Comments

However the material recovered from a digital device is used, it is highly likely that it will have some value as part of an intelligence gathering/

profiling exercise, and it has been suggested that some form of "judicial wiretapping" as already used in Germany and Austria [1, 14] may be desirable in order to secure concrete evidence of criminal acts. The counter-argument to this is that lawful use of viral/Trojan/worm software creates new opportunities for unlawful use of the same software. It is not hard to envision a situation where a criminal obtains a copy of "judicial malware" and subverts it to their own purposes.

Many investigators have formed the opinion that, no matter what type of enquiry they have been asked to conduct, they will encounter material which is indicative of inolvement in other crimes at some stage of their work. In these cases, a decision needs to be taken – what should be done with this extra material ?

Clearly, if the evidence gathered indicates that the person under investigation may have been involved in more serious crime, then it must be passed to the appropriate bodies for further investigation. However, if the evidence is less obvious, giving just a general impression of criminality, legal boundaries and ethics must be considered.

Whatever the situation is, though, digital evidence is with us to stay, and its utility in any investigation seems set to increase.

10
Case Studies and Examples

10.1 Introduction

This chapter aims to give you, the reader, a chance to see and practice the application of the techniques and methods described in the preceding chapters.

Some of the cases presented here are real, but anonymised as much as possible to avoid causing further distress to those directly involved, others are fictitious but based on typical cases in which the author has been involved.

10.2 Copyright violation

As we saw in Chapter 2, modern technology has made it very easy for anyone to copy or produce CDs and DVDs without the permission of the copyright owners.

UK copyright agencies such as the MCPS-PRS alliance, FACT and the BPI, working with Trading Standards Departments, police and other agencies, regularly investigate and prosecute those involved. Whether those under investigation are working alone, or are part of organised crime is a subject of some debate but, no matter who they are, all investigations typically follow the same path.

Digital Forensics: Digital Evidence in Criminal Investigation   Angus M. Marshall
© 2008 John Wiley & Sons, Ltd

Firstly, a complaint of copyright violation will be received. On its own, this it not sufficient to allow a full investigation to proceed, but is often followed-up by an agent of the copyright holder making a "test purchase". Here, they act the part of an ordinary customer buying one or more of the alleged "fakes" from the suspect. Once they have received their goods, either in person at something like a car-boot sale, or through the post as a result of online sales, the received goods are checked for similarity to material which is subject to copyright or other protection in law.

If it can be established, at this stage, that the material supplied has been produced without the copyright-owner's permission, a warrant is requested to allow search of the suspect's premises and seizure of equipment relating to the suspected offence.

Any seizure will, of course, comply with prevailing guidelines (See Chapter 3) to ensure that there can be no allegations of contamination.

We know, from Chapter 2, that computer equipment in these cases falls into the "Tool" category, but also has some roles as "Witness" and "Guardian". Each of these categories allows us to identify the type of evidence which we might find on a suspect's PC.

Firstly, let us consider the "Guardianship" role. Primarily, this applies to DVDs which are equipped with region codes and encryption to prevent, or least discourage, copying. In order to bypass these copy-protection systems, the computer must have been equipped with additional software to allow not just playback, but copying. Therefore, the presence of DVD-decryption software is an indication that the machine may have been used for the production of illegal copies. Furthermore, if we can show that the DVD-decryption software was used at the same time that files representing the contents of a DVD appeared on the machine in question, then we have a strong indication that a user of the machine chose to copy the DVD contents, making it a "Knowing Authorised" act (see Chapter 5).

A collection of files, representing the contents of several different discs, could then be taken as an indication that it was very likely that all of these files had been created through the use of DVD-decryption software.

Added to the data files, we typically check for the presence of cover artwork and disc labels, either produced by scanning the originals or by downloading from one of the web sites which specialise in making these available. Whichever method is used, the presence of these files is almost always an indication of another series of "Knowing Authorised" acts where the computer is acting as a "Tool".

Next, we would look for evidence of manufacture. Apart from possession of a large quantity of blank discs, we seek to determine if the suspect is in possession of any "home-made" discs. If he/she has multiple copies, it is usually an indication of intent to supply or trade.

If we can also show, through examination of log files, deleted files and temporary files, that some or all of the data files on the storage device have been written to DVD or CD, and that those DVDs or CDs match the ones in the suspect's possession or which were supplied during the test purchase, then we have something close to conclusive proof that the machine has been used to manufacture illegal copies.

Finally, we consider the computer's role as "Witness", and other activities such as e-mail and use of WWW sites (e.g. online auctions, chatrooms etc.), financial record keeping, printing of mailing labels and posters, phone calls, text messages and instant messenger services, which would provide additional confirmation that the suspect has been trading.

10.2.1 Real case: the auto-maintenance bookshop

One of the author's early copyright-violation investigations dealt with someone who was allegedly selling copies of motor maintenance manuals on an auction site. Not only did the hard disc of the suspect's computer contain complete copies of each manual that had been sold, but it also contained cached copies of the auction pages created by the suspect, and a spreadsheet containing the name, address, e-mail address, phone number, product, amount paid and status of feedback for each purchaser. In effect, the perpetrator's obsessive record keeping had created a full confession, which the computer had witnessed.

10.3 Missing person and murder

In a missing persons case, we usually consider digital devices' roles as witnesses first. Our objective is twofold. Firstly, we want to determine the last time that the missing person was actively using a device, to corroborate a witness statement or provide evidence of their location at a later time than a human witness can provide. Secondly, we look for any evidence of communications indicating a threat to the missing person, or previously unknown plans to meet someone.

The first of our goals can be achieved by use of timeline analysis (see Chapters 4, 6, 8 and 9). Careful examination of the timestamps on data held on the device can provide us with an indication of when any activity occurred, while examination of the data gives a good insight into the nature of the activity.

Our second goal requires a more detailed analysis of data held on the device. Following correct examination procedures (Chapters 4 and 8) we attempt to recover as much data as possible. Analysis of the material recovered may give us access to copies of e-mails, SMS messages, chatroom sessions etc. showing that the missing person has been the victim of bullying, paedophilic grooming or some other activity which has led to them going to a secret meeting or similar.

If we are unable to recover the missing person's mobile phone, interrogation of the network may allow us to find their current location or, at least, the location in which their phone was switched off. Use of credit/debit cards, travel passes, loyalty cards etc. may allow us to build up a pattern of movement or activity too.

10.3.1 Real case: where has she gone?

The author was contacted by a police force to assist with a missing person enquiry. Although the force in question had its own high-tech crime unit, the unit was over-loaded with other urgent casework and could not assist as quickly as the investigating team wanted.

A young woman (A) had gone missing sometime between breakfast and early evening on a Friday (let's say it was the 6th of June). Her partner (B) had last seen her at home and had had no contact with her since. The woman was known to have been working on her home computer because her aunt had exchanged e-mails with her during the morning, but the woman had not been seen since.

The questions which needed immediate answers were:

- When was the last activity on the computer that could have been carried out by the missing person?

- Was any of the activity carried out after the last e-mail was sent?

- Was there anything to suggest she had arranged to meet someone?

- Was there anything else of significance on the computer?

Examination of the hard disc produced cached copies of web pages from the webmail system which A had been using. These corroborated the times from her aunt's received e-mails and showed that A had been using the home computer at the times in question. There was no indication of e-mail or other communications with any other person after the last e-mail to her mother.

Further examination produced a timeline showing that A had carried on working, using a word processor, for about another 15 minutes before the computer was shut down. Thus, the computer was the only witness to those 15 minutes of activity.

Later the same day, the computer was clearly switched on again and used to access more web pages. B confirmed that he had come home and had been searching for CDs in online shops. Again, the cached web pages corroborated this.

Unfortunately, during the examination of the computer, A's body was found, and the missing person enquiry escalated into a murder investigation.

B was under suspicion following the old principle that murder is more likely to be committed by someone close to the victim than a complete stranger.

Mobile phone evidence led the investigating team to believe that the murder had happened some time on the Friday, and they wanted to know if B could have had the opportunity to get home, kill A and return to work without anyone noticing. Because B had been alone in his office, their initial thinking was that he would have had plenty of time.

Modified	Accessed	Created
06-06-2008 12:35:43	09-06-2008	09-06-2008 11:07:19

Figure 10.1 Suspicious file properties

During examination of the hard disc a file with unusual properties had been noticed (Figure 10.1).

The file in question seemed to have been created on the Monday (9th June)*AFTER* it was last modified.

In a situation such as this, the first thought is naturally that someone has changed the clock on the computer in an attempt to hide the real time and date when they were really using the machine. If this is done, though, it usually results in several files having inconsistent timestamps. Here, there was only a single file.

The search for an explanation of these strange file properties led to a hypothesis: could Windows be recording the time that the file first appeared on the machine, but maintaining the time when it was last modified somewhere else?

Some experimental work with the same version of Windows as A's PC soon showed that our hypothesis was correct. Whenever a file was copied from one machine onto a floppy disc and onto a second machine, the second machine gave the file a new creation timestamp: the time it first appeared on that machine. The other timestamps didn't change.

Inspection of the content of the file showed that it was something that B had been working on in his office on the Friday. By mid-morning on Monday he was so concerned about A's disappearance that he couldn't carry on working in his office and had decided to go home. Being conscientious, though, he had decided to take some work home with him and, fortunately, the file in question was the one he had been working on around the time of the disappearance.

The suspicious file on the home PC turned out to provide B with an alibi. The computers were acting as witnesses, proving that he had been at work around the time of the disappearance and could not have returned home in time to murder A.

10.4 The view of a defence witness

To many, a defence witness is "the enemy" – a hired gun whose sole purpose is to use "smoke and mirrors" to destroy the prosecution case. Although there may be a few "experts" who work in this way,[1] the greater majority are professionals who work to the same standards, and to answer the same questions, as the experts for the other side. True expert witnesses know that they are responsible to the court and have a duty to present the truth as they find it. They have a duty to explore reasonable explanations for the material recovered and to scrutinise the prosecution reports independently, in accordance with ACPO Principle 3 (Chapter 3 [2]).

In some cases this may mean that they have to report failings in processes or procedures or give alternate explanations, at other times they find themselves agreeing with the prosecution expert.

It is not unknown for a defence expert to recover more evidence of guilt than the prosecution have chosen to present. In this situation, some lengthy discussions with the legal team often lead to a recommendation that the client should plead guilty in order to avoid a long and costly trial which will ultimately result in that verdict anyway.

10.4.1 Real case: fraud prosecution failure

One case in which the author was involved was a private prosecution dealing with allegations of financial irregularity. A company director, who had recently taken control of a company, was accusing previous directors of false accounting and fraud. A significant part of the case revolved around letters which, the new director alleged, had been sent by one of the previous directors without the knowledge of anyone in the company and which indicated that some tax calculations were being carried out improperly.

The author was asked, by the defence solicitor, to examine the allegations contained in the prosecution material and comment on the validity of evidence derived from the main computer in the company.

---

[1] Usually they can be identified by the presence of cowboy hats and spurs.

It very quickly became apparent that there was a problem.

During the takeover period, the main server for the company had developed a fault and been sent for repair. After two or three weeks of maintenance, using normal maintenance software, the computer had been returned to the new director, who had kept it in his possession and allowed a friend to examine it, before handing it over to a professional forensic computing firm for full examination. The firm in question was not fully aware of what had happened to the machine prior to their involvement and it only became completely apparent during defence enquiries.

Thus, there was a four week period when the computer's history was not fully documented (violating ACPO Principle 3). In addition to this, the maintenance process had caused huge changes to the state of the hard disc, which could not be fully explained by any of the people who had accessed it during the four-week period (violating ACPO Principles 1 and 2). In short, the evidence recovered from the computer could not be considered wholly reliable because it had been mishandled. In particular, the week when it was in the possession of the new director had created an opportunity where someone directly involved in the case could have deliberately manipulated and altered the data to make their evidence appear stronger.

If the prosecution team had handed the computer over to the forensic computing firm earlier in the process, it would have been much harder to suggest that there was any opportunity for irregularity in the recovered material.

Even if the inherent reliability of the data recovered, based on timestamps etc., was not open to challenge, there was an additional confounding factor. The server in question was running an old version of Microsoft Windows which had neither strong security nor proper auditing features present. As a result, there was a flaw in the Infrastructure/Organisation/Activities/Procedures components of the system (see Chapter 5) which allowed the entities to alter data without it being properly controlled and recorded. As a result, even if we could say *when* evidential material appeared on the system it would have been impossible to trace its origin completely.

Ultimately, when the case eventually got to court, the prosecution presented no evidence and the defendant was acquitted with costs awarded against the private prosecutor.

If nothing else, this case highlights the importance of establishing and maintaining continuity of evidence by using correct procedures from the outset.

Appendix A
The "Aircraft Carrier" PC

Further images of the "aircraft carrier" PC, courtesy of
http://www.mini-itx.com/.[1]

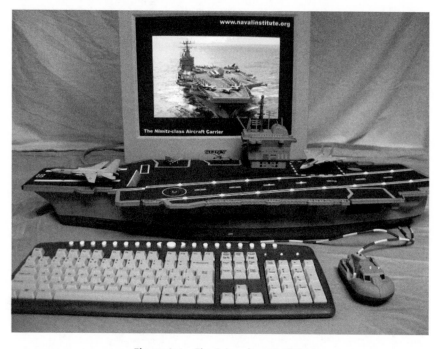

Figure A.1 The "aircraft carrier" PC

---

[1]Images are copyright www.mini-itx.com and reproduced by permission.

Digital Forensics: Digital Evidence in Criminal Investigation   Angus M. Marshall
© 2008 John Wiley & Sons, Ltd

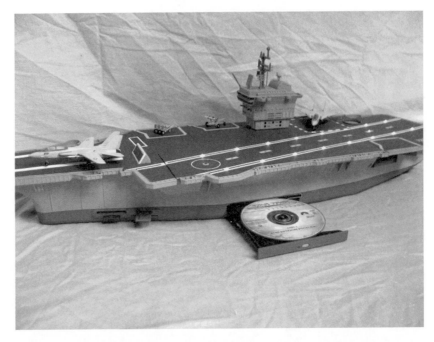

Figure A.2   Detail showing the DVD-rewriter drawer extended

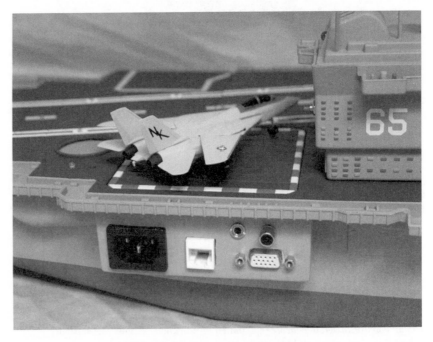

Figure A.3   Connectors on the "rear"

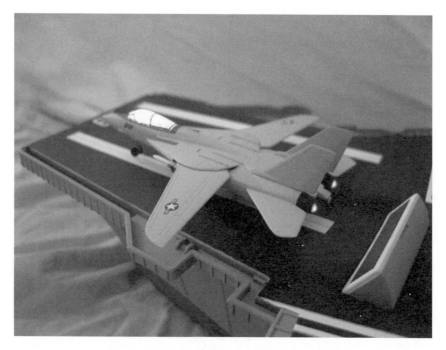

Figure A.4 Activity lights in aircraft on carrier deck

Appendix B
Additional Resources

This is by no means a comprehensive list of all tools, but is intended to give brief information about the most commonly encountered tools used in investigations.

B.1 Hard disc and storage laboratory tools

- EnCase by Guidance Software is the most popular digital evidence tool in use worldwide at the time of writing. It exists in several different forms, but has been adopted as standard by most law-enforcement organisations. [Commercial]

- Forensic ToolKit (FTK) by AccessData has just undergone a major revision from version 1.71 to version 2. V1.71 was somewhat limited in functionality compared to EnCase, but V2 seems to address many of these issues. [Commercial]

- SMART from ASR Data differs from EnCase and FTK in that it runs on Linux rather than Windows. It has similar features to both FTK and EnCase and is a fairly popular alternative for those who prefer to use Linux as their main operating system. [Commercial]

- Sleuthkit and Autopsy by Brian Carrier. These tools have grown out of the older "Coroner's Toolkit" package which was developed by @stake. As

Digital Forensics: Digital Evidence in Criminal Investigation Angus M. Marshall
© 2008 John Wiley & Sons, Ltd

two open-source projects (Sleuthkit is a set of tools for data extraction, Autopsy is the web-based interface), they offer a powerful free alternative to the commercial products, with an emphasis on post-incident diagnostics. [Open source/free.]

B.2 Mobile phone/PDA tools

- .XRY from MicroSystemation AB is a combination of hardware interface plus software for data extraction. [Commercial]

- CellDek, developed by the UK Forensic Science Service and marketed by LogiCube, consists of a specialised hardware interface module with a selection of interface leads and specialist software for data extraction. [Commercial]

- Device Seizure by Paraben consists of a hardware pack containing interface leads, a SIM card reader and specialist software to extract data from a wide range of handsets. [Commercial.]

B.3 Live CDs

- HELIX: based on Linux, this includes a selection of incident response and analysis tools, including Sleuthkit and Autopsy. It can be run on top of Windows for live analysis and imaging, or can be used as a boot disc to perform offline imaging from the suspect machine. [Open source/free]

- BackTrack2 is similar to HELIX, but the toolset is focussed more on network analysis than on data extraction and analysis. [Open source/free.]

B.4 Recommended reading

The following books are amongst the most useful for anyone starting out in Digital Forensics work:

- *Incident Response: Computer Forensics Toolkit* by Douglas Schweizer. Publisher: John Wiley & Sons, Ltd, 2003

- *Computer Forensics JumpStart* by Michael Solomon, Diane Barrett and Neil Broom. Publisher: John Wiley & Sons, Ltd, 2004

- *Handbook of Computer Crime Investigation: Forensic Tools and Technology* by Eoghan Casey. Publisher: Academic Press, 2001

- *Digital Evidence and Computer Crime* (2nd ed.) by Eoghan Casey. Publisher: Academic Press, 2004

- *Investigating Child Exploitation and Pornography: The Internet, Law and Forensic Science* by Monique Ferraro and Eoghan Casey. Publisher: Academic Press, 2004.

- *File System Forensic Analysis* by Brian Carrier. Publisher: Pearson Education, 2005.

- *Windows Forensics: The Field Guide for Corporate Computer Investigations* by Chad Steel. Publisher: John Wiley & Sons, Ltd, 2006.

Appendix C
SIM Card Data Report

This is a sample report produced using the Netherlands Forensic Institute's
TULP2G free software.

Digital Forensics: Digital Evidence in Criminal Investigation   Angus M. Marshall
© 2008 John Wiley & Sons, Ltd

☑ Show case data ☑ Show documentation ☐ Show "preformatted" SMS text

Netherlands Forensic Institute - TULP2G

Case name	Ruby Slippers
Case creator	C. Lion
Creation date	23/01/2008 14:52:36
MD5 hash	CC6C871C0399796D6E5FEE10DF5F5306
SHA-1 hash	E765A4BBD04B9F1064BBA510E739CBF11966A140

Notes

This is an example case with settings for the examination of SIM cards.

Go to the Investigation tab for reading the SIM.

Plug-in info

Plug-in type	Plug-in info
ExportPlugin	TULP2G.Export.XML, Version=1.3.0.4, Culture=neutral, PublicKeyToken=3480a3624ac48f93
ConversionPlugin	TULP2G.Conversion.SIM, Version=1.3.0.5, Culture=neutral, PublicKeyToken=3480a3624ac48f93
ConversionPlugin	TULP2G.Conversion.SMS, Version=1.3.0.3, Culture=neutral, PublicKeyToken=3480a3624ac48f93

Investigation *Ruby Slippers*

Investigator	C. Lion
Creation date	23/01/2008 14:52:36
MD5 hash	EDCB64BF9D789B2021A71289FDE0CBC9
SHA-1 hash	3DE3183C447D2A3BC8E5D6CAF270141429EB0823
MD5 SIM hash	04DB1551F9EFAB0A34F8CDE751DDF7C3
SHA-1 SIM hash	B84C0D0B598F154746A1DA367DA6C9ABA505D319

Notes

Select the "Configure..." button next to the Protocol Plug-in for reading the PIN- and PUK status and PIN or PUK entry.

After correct PIN/PUK entry the SIM can be read by selecting the "Run" button. If the SIM can't be read, then change the "Disable PTS" setting in the configuration screen of the Communication Plug-in.

After the SIM has been read, a report can be made by selecting the "Run" button from the "Report" tab.

Plug-in info

Plug-in type	Plug-in info

ProtocolPlugin	TULP2G.Protocol.ProtocolSIM@TULP2G.Protocol.SIM, Version=1.3.0.6, Culture=neutral, PublicKeyToken=3480a3624ac48f93
CommunicationPlugin	TULP2G.Communication.PCSC@TULP2G.Communication.PCSC, Version=1.3.0.2, Culture=neutral, PublicKeyToken=3480a3624ac48f93

☑ Card Holder Verification (CHV)

Data in a Subscriber Identity Module (SIM) can be protected with PINs (Personal Identity Numbers). A PIN consists of four to eight digits, is requested after a phone has been switched on, and can be entered using the phone's keyboard. The number of attempts to enter a PIN is limited to three. If none of the attempts is successful, access to the protected data will be blocked. This block can be cancelled with a PUK (PIN unblocking code). A PUK consists of eight digits and includes a new PIN. The number of attempts to enter a PUK is limited to ten. If none of the attempts is successful, the possibility to cancel the PIN block will be disabled permanently. The Card Holder Verification (CHV) table lists all CHV operations in chronological order done during the examination. There are two types of operations:

Verification
*   The verified PIN and or PUK code(s)*
Status
*   The actual number of attempts left and the enabled/disabled state of the code (only for PIN).*

	PIN	PUK	PIN2	PUK2
Status	3 (disabled)	10	3	10
Status	3 (disabled)	10	3	10

☑ Integrated Circuit Card (ICC) identification

A unique identification number for the SIM. Content is defined in CCITT Recomendation E.118 which defines a major industry identifier (89), a country code, an issuer identifier and a individual account identification number. CCITT stands for Comité Consultatif International Téléphonique et Télégraphique, an organization that sets international communications standards.

8944302700816199999 (United Kingdom)

☑ International Mobile Subscriber Indentity (IMSI)

A unique identification number within the complete GSM network. This number consists of a country code, a network provider code and a subscriber number.

234907859399299 (United Kingdom, T-Mobile UK)

☑ SIM service table

This table sums up all the services that can be supported by a SIM. Under allocated an indication is given of whether or not each service can be supported by the card; whether or not a service has been activated can be found under activated. All services in this list can be stored in a SIM

Nr.	Description	Allocated	Activated
0	CHV1 disable function	■	■
1	Fixed Dialling Numbers (FDN)	■	■
2	no description available	■	☐
3	Short Message Storage (SMS)	■	■
4	Advice of Charge (AoC)	☐	☐

Netherlands Forensic Institute – TULP2G Report   12/06/2008 18:39

5	Capability Configuration Parameters (CCP)	■	■
6	PLMN selector	■	■
7	RFU	□	□
8	MSISDN	■	■
9	Extension1	■	■
10	Extension2	□	□
11	SMS Parameters	■	■
12	Last Number Dialled (LND)	□	□
13	Cell Broadcast Message Identifier	□	□
14	Group Identifier Level 1	■	■
15	Group Identifier Level 2	□	□
16	Service Provider Name	■	■
17	Service Dialling Numbers (SDN)	□	□
18	Extension3	□	□
19	RFU	□	□
20	VGCS Group Identifier List (EFvgcs and EFvgcss)	□	□
21	VBS Group Identifier List (EFvbs and EFvbss)	□	□
22	enhanced Multi-Level Precedence and Pre-emption Service	□	□
23	Automatic Answer for eMLPP	□	□
24	Data download via SMS-CB	□	□
25	Data download via SMS-PP	■	■
26	Menu selection	■	■
27	Call control	□	□
28	Proactive SIM	■	■
29	Cell Broadcast Message Identifier Ranges	□	□
30	Barred Dialling Numbers (BDN)	□	□
31	Extension4	□	□
32	De-personalization Control Keys	□	□
33	Co-operative Network List	□	□
34	Show Message Status Reports	□	□
35	Network's indication of alerting in the MS	□	□
36	Mobile Originated Short Message control by SIM	□	□
37	GPRS	□	□
38	Image (IMG)	■	■
39	SoLSA (Support of Local Service Area)	□	□
40	USSD string data object supported in Call Control	□	□
41	RUN AT COMMAND command	□	□
42	PLMN Selector List with Access Technology	□	□
43	OPLMN Seleclor List with Access Technology	□	□
44	HPLMN Access Technology	□	□
45	CPBCCH Information	□	□
46	Investigation Scan	□	□
47	Extended Capability Configuration Parameters	□	□

☑ Service Provider Name (SPN)

Name of the service provider, with a field indicating whether the registered network should be shown on the display of the phone.

(display of registered PLMN required)

☑ Subscriber dialling numbers

Names and phone numbers, to be entered by the user, intended for storing the subscriber's own numbers. The first number is often shown on the display of the GSM telephone when it is switched on. Other numbers that might be shown include fax and data numbers.

Pos.	Name	Number
1		07847470636

☑ Abbreviated dialling numbers

Names and phone numbers, to be entered and changed by the subscriber, which can be chosen easily using the phone. Recovered number data is shown in italics. For long numbers a "...[4]" indicates that the rest of the number is stored in the "4th" position of the "Extension1" file.

Pos.	Name	Number
1	Tinman	070xxxxxxxx
2	Scarecrow	078xxxxxxxx

☑ Fixed dialling numbers

Names and phone numbers, to be entered and changed by the subscriber, which can be chosen easily using the phone. A phone can be configured in such a way that only phone numbers from this list can be called. This list can only be adjusted by means of a second PIN code. Recovered number data is shown in italics. For long numbers a "...[4]" indicates that the rest of the number is stored in the "4th" position of the "Extension2" file.

☑ Language preference

This list, entered by the card supplier and to be adjusted by the subscriber, indicates the subscriber's language preferences in descending priority. This preference can be used by the GSM telephone for selecting display texts in the correct language.

Priority	Coding group	Language	Coding	Message class	Compression
1	0 (Language using the default alphabet)	1 (English)			

☑ Public Land Mobile Network (PLMN) selector

When a phone cannot find its own network, for instance because the phone is abroad, the phone will start searching for other GSM networks. This searching takes place in the order of the list shown. In this way network providers, and also subscribers, can specify their preference for networks to be used when the phone is outside the range of its own network.

Priority	Country	Network
1	228 (Switzerland)	01 (Swisscom GSM)
2	208 (France)	10 (S.F.R.)
3	262 (Germany)	03 (E-Plus Mobilfunk GmbH & Co. KG)

☑ Home PLMN (HPLMN) search period

The interval in minutes during which a phone should search for its own network. This searching takes place when the phone is in the country of the subscriber, but is connected to a different (competing) network.

255 (1530 minutes)

☑ Forbidden PLMNs

This list consists of GSM networks that may not be selected automatically by the phone for establishing a connection. A network may be included in this list because this information has been added to the SIM by the subscriber's network provider or because the network with which the GSM telephone tried to establish a connection refuses this connection. When a new, refusing network should be added to a full list, the element which has been in the list longest (first position) will be erased. The new refusing network appears as the last item on the list. A subscriber may force an attempt to establish contact with a network from this list manually via the phone. If this attempt is successful, the network will be removed from the list.

Position	Country	Network
1	234 (United Kingdom)	33 (Orange)
2	234 (United Kingdom)	15 (Vodafone Ltd)
3	234 (United Kingdom)	10 (O2 UK Ltd)

☑ Location information

A GSM network consists of cells which are responsible for radio communications between mobile phones and the network. A number of cells are grouped together in local areas. Each phone keeps the network informed about the local area where the phone is. In this way, the network can establish contact with a GSM subscriber by sending a search signal to all the cells in the local area where the GSM telephone is. The following information regarding the most recent local area is stored in the SIM:

TIMSI
> *A temporary IMSI which is adjusted each time the local area changes. This is done to make sure that subscribers cannot be traced on the basis of the IMSI.*

Update timer
> *This value indicates how often a phone should inform the network of the current local area. This data is used only in Phase 1 SIMs.*

Update status
> *The status of the transfer of location information.*

MCC
> *The country where the local area is situated.*

MNC
> *The network of which the local area forms part.*

LAC
> *A reference to the local area itself.*

TIMSI	Update timer	Update status
0xFFFFFFFF	15	not_updated
Local Area Information		
MCC	MNC	LAC
234 (United Kingdom)	30 (T-Mobile UK)	0xFFFE

☑ Broadcast control channels

Netherlands Forensic Institute – TULP2G Report   12/06/2008 18:39

Broadcast control channels are communication channels to which all inactive phones respond in order to determine which cell from which network would be optimum for communication. The intention of this data is to simplify this selection process. Although not clearly specified, this list should contain the neigbouring cell frequencies broadcasted by the last cell of the home PLMN on which the phone camped.

0xBB1D99E34B866897F4F36F3A83E4DB78

☑ Short Message Service (SMS) parameters

Parameters that can be used by the GSM telephone for outgoing SMS messages. Each parameter consists of the following elements:

Position
 Storage position of the parameter set.
Name
 (Optional) text describing the set.
TP-DestinationAddress
 Number of a recipient (usually left blank, as this normally differs for each message).
TP-ServiceCentreAddress
 Number of a service centre where the messages are processed.
TP-ValidityPeriod
 The period of validity of a message. When a message has been sent but the recipient cannot be contacted, the service centre may decide, after the period of validity has lapsed, not to make any further attempts to deliver the message.

Position	Name	Destination Address	Service Centre Address	Validity Period
1			+447958879890	3 Days

☑ SMS status

An internal reference to the most recent outgoing SMS and an indication of the availability of SIM memory for storing messages, so that the GSM network can be informed as soon as memory is available.

Last transfer layer protocol message reference: 0, memory capacity exceeded: no.

☑ SMS messages

Messages which can be received and sent with a mobile phone. The messages can also be sent in a different way: e.g. via the Internet or by telephoning a special number and recording a message, which is then converted into text and sent as an SMS message to a mobile phone. Below is an explanation of possible message elements.

Position
 Storage position of the message.
Ext. type
 Type of message according to the phone.
Int. type
 Type of message according to the SMS decoder.
Part
 One storage position might be part of a larger message.
Timestamp
 Date and time when the message was received at the service centre. The date is shown as ◆month-day-year◆; the time is the local time at the service centre, followed by the number of hours of difference in comparison with Greenwich Mean Time. For messages of type REPORT the timestamp identifies the time when the service centre received the message related to the report.

Discharge timestamp
Parameter identifying the time associated with a particular status outcome.
Validity Period
When a message has been sent but the recipient cannot be contacted, the service centre may decide, after the period of validity has elapsed, not to make any further attempts to deliver the message.
Service Centre address
Number of the service centre where the messages is processed.
Originating address
Number of the sender.
Destination address
Number of the recipient.

Nr.	Ext. Type	Int. Type	Part	Timestamp
1	read	TextMessageType	All/1	07-12-07 10:18:19 GMT
Service Centre Address			**Originating Address**	
+447958879884			+4478xxxxxxxx	
Content				
RS has left OZ. Meet at Emerald castle at 12				

References

[1] W. Abel. Trojans, agents and tags: The next generation of investigators, *BILETA Conference*, 2008.

[2] ACPO, The Association of Chief Police Officers. *Good Practice Guide for Computer Based Electronic Evidence V4.0*. ACPO/7safe, 2007.
Online: http://www.7safe.com/electronic-evidence/.

[3] F. Anklesaria, M. McCahill, P. Lindner *et al.* RFC1436: The Internet Gopher Protocol (a distributed document search and retrieval protocol). *Internet RFCs*, 1993.

[4] T. Bardin. *Bootstrapping: Douglas Englebart, Coevolution and the Origins of Personal Computing*, pages 38–42. Stanford University Press, Stanford, CA, USA, 2000.

[5] T. Berners-Lee. Information management: A proposal. *CERN internal publication*, 1989.
Online: http://www.w3.org/History/1989/proposal.html/

[6] Bluetooth Special Interest Group. Bluetooth.com.
Online: http://www. bluetooth.com/

[7] D. Canter. *Criminal Shadows: Inside the Mind of the Serial Killer*. Harper Collins, London, 1995.

[8] J. Chposky and T. Leonsis. *Blue Magic: the People, the Power and the Politics behind the IBM Personal Computer*. Grafton, London, 1989.

[9] R. V. Clarke and M. Felson (eds.). *Routine Activity and Rational Choice. Advances in Criminological Theory*, volume 5. Transaction Books, New Brunswick, NJ, USA, 1993.

[10] L. E. Cohen and M. Felson. Social change and crime rate trends: a routine activity approach. *American Sociological Review*, 44:588–608, 1979.

[11] N. Cohen and K. Maclennan-Brown. *Digital Imaging Procedure V2.0*. Home Office Scientific Development Branch, November 2007.

[12] M. Crispin. RFC3501: Internet message access protocol – version 4rev1. *Internet RFCs*, 2003.

[13] D. H. Crocker. RFC822: Standard for ARPA internet text messages. *Internet RFCs*, 1982.

[14] M. Damm. I know what you saved last summer! – the use of secret spy software by crime investigators. *BILETA Conference*, 2008.

[15] ECMA. Standard ECMA-376, office open xml file formats, 2006.
Online: http://www.ecma-international.org/publications/standards/Ecma-376.htm

[16] W. Gibson. *Neuromancer*. Ace, New York, USA, 1984.

[17] R. Gordon. *Doctor in the House*. Joseph, London, 1952.

[18] GSM Association. GSM world.
Online: http://www.gsmworld.com/.

[19] J. A. Halderman, S. Schoen, N. Heninger *et al.* Lest we remember: Cold boot attacks on encryption keys, 2008.
Online: http://citp.princeton.edu/ memory.

[20] P. Hayes. No sorry from lovebug author. *The Register*, 2005.
Online: http:// www.theregister.co.uk/2005/05/11/love_bug_author/.

[21] HM Government. Regulation of Investigatory Powers Act. 2000.
Online: http://www.opsi.gov.uk/acts/acts2000/ukpga_20000023_en_1.

[22] D. A. Huffman. A method for the construction of minimum redundancy codes. *Proceedings of the Institute of Radio Engineers*, 40:1098–1101, 1952.

[23] IEEE. IEEE802.11, The working group setting the standards for wireless LAN.
Online: http://www.ieee802.org/11/.

[24] ISO (International Standards Organization). ISO/IEC 7498-1:1994 *Open Systems Interconnection Model*, 1994.

[25] A. M. Marshall. Digital evidence, *Measurement and Control*, 38 (3):79–82, 2005.

[26] A. M. Marshall and B. Gwynne. The application of crimelites to examination of computer components 'in situ'. *Science and Justice*, 45:151–155, 2005.

[27] A. M. Marshall and B. C. Tompsett. Spam 'n' chips – a discussion of internet crime. *Science and Justice*, 42:117–122, April–June, 2002.

[28] A. M. Marshall and B. C. Tompsett. Silicon pathology. *Science and Justice*, 44:43–50, January-March, 2004.

[29] A. M. Marshall and B. C. Tompsett. Identity theft in an online world. *Computer Law and Security Report*, 21(2):128–137, 2005.

[30] A. M. Marshall, G. Moore, and B. C. Tompsett. Criminalisation of the internet: an examination of illegal activity online. In *EAFS 2006*, 2006.

[31] R. C. Merkle. A fast software one-way hash function. *The Journal of Cryptology*, 3(1):43–58, 1989.

[32] G. Moore. Cramming more components onto integrated circuits. *Electronics*, 38(8):114–117, 1965.

[33] Moving Picture Experts Group. MPEG home page.
Online: http://www.chiariglione.org/mpeg/.

[34] J. Myers and M. Rose. RFC1939: Post office protocol – version 3. *Internet RFCs*, 1996.

[35] T. Nelson. *Computers, Creativity and the Nature of the Written Word*. Lecture given at Vassar College, New York, USA, 1965.

[36] NIST (The National Institute of Standards). *Secure Hash Standard (SHA-1). Standard 180-1*. Available online at http://www.itl.nist.gov/ fipspubs/fip180-1.htm (last viewed 31st January 2005).

[37] OASIS Open Document Technical Committee. Oasis open document format for office applications (opendocument).
Online: http://www.oasisopen.org/committees/tc_home.php?wg_abbrev=office.

[38] E. A. Poe. *The Purloined Letter*, 1844.

[39] J. B. Postel. RFC821: Simple mail transfer protocol. *Internet RFCs*, 1982.

[40] W. Rankl and W. Effing. *Smart Card Handbook*, 4th edition. John Wiley & Sons, Ltd, Chichester, UK, 2003.

[41] J. K. Reynolds. RFC918: Post office protocol. *Internet RFCs*, 1984.

[42] R. L. Rivest. RFC1321, the MD5 message-digest algorithm. *Internet RFCs*, 1992.

[43] L. Roberts. Multiple computer networks and intercomputer communication. *ACM Gatlinburg Conference*, 1967.

[44] S. Singh. *The Code Book*. Fourth Estate, London, 2000.

[45] E. H. Spafford. The internet wormd program: An analysis, 1988.
Online: http://homes.cerias.purdue.edu/spaf/tech-reps/823. pdf.

[46] F. Tipton. *Information Security Management Handbook*, 6th edition. Auerbach, 2007.

[47] B. C. Tompsett and A. M. Marshall. Holistic information security. *Cyberprofiling Project Research Report*, Universities of Hull and Teesside, 2004.

[48] B. C. Tompsett, A. M. Marshall, and N. C. Semmens. Cyberprofiling. In *Computer Network Forensics Research Workshop*, IEEE. Athens, Greece, 2005.

[49] Unicode Inc. Unicode home page.
Online: http://unicode.org/.

[50] USB Implementers' Forum. Universal serial bus mass storage class implementation overview, 2003.
Online: http://www.usb.org/developers/devclass_docs/usb_msc_overview1.2.pdf.

[51] W3C (World Wide Web Consortium). Exensible markup language (XML). 1996-2003.
Online: http://www.w3.org/XML/.

[52] S. Walklate. *Handbook of Victims and Victimology*. Willan Publishing, 2007.

[53] J. Ziv and A. Lempel. A universal algorithm for sequential data compression. *IEEE Transactions on Information Theory*, 23:337–342, 1977.

Index